# Endorsements

"Having had personal experience with a bone marrow disorder with my husband, the late Congressman Bob Matsui, I believe that anyone who has lived with someone with a life-threatening illness will benefit from Rusty Hammer's words and wisdom. As a patient, advocate, and leader, Rusty has seen these challenges from all sides. His journey provides lessons that can help both those who are afflicted and their families."

   —**Congresswoman Doris O. Matsui**, Sacramento, California

"Through his insightful and heartfelt descriptions of his experiences with a dreaded disease, Rusty not only teaches us much about medicine, but in the end about humanity. I am honored to care for him and learn from him."

   —**Robert S. Negrin, MD,** Division Chief, Bone Marrow
   Transplant, Stanford Hospital and Medical Center

"Rusty Hammer's description of his journey to overcome leukemia will inspire all who face the difficult and life-changing presence of a cancer diagnosis. His insights, and the thoughtful way he has expressed himself, will make patients feel less alone and more hopeful, and physicians who read it will take better care of those patients for whom the call is yet to come."

**—Stephen J. Forman, MD,**
City of Hope Bone Marrow Division

# When Cancer Calls ...
# Say Yes to Life

# ALSO BY RUSSELL J. HAMMER

The Business Perspective: 2002–2006
Exploring Los Angeles Public Policy Issues Through the Lens of Business

# When Cancer Calls ...
# Say Yes to Life

## The Story of One Man's Journey through Leukemia

### Rusty Hammer

iUniverse, Inc.
New York Lincoln Shanghai

# When Cancer Calls … Say Yes to Life
## The Story of One Man's Journey through Leukemia

iUniverse books may be ordered through booksellers or by contacting:

iUniverse
2021 Pine Lake Road, Suite 100
Lincoln, NE 68512
www.iuniverse.com
1-800-Authors (1-800-288-4677)

Because of the dynamic nature of the Internet, any Web addresses or links contained in this book may have changed since publication and may no longer be valid.

The information, ideas, and suggestions in this book are not intended as a substitute for professional medical advice. Before following any suggestions contained in this book, you should consult your personal physician. Neither the author nor the publisher shall be liable or responsible for any loss or damage allegedly arising as a consequence of your use or application of any information or suggestions in this book.

Original Cover Artwork by Megan J. Hackard
Photo on page 53 by Marlee Miller
Illustration on page 221 by Lisa Ferdinansen

ISBN: 978-0-595-44735-0 (pbk)
ISBN: 978-0-595-69071-8 (cloth)
ISBN: 978-0-595-89056-9 (ebk)

Printed in the United States of America

Webster's defines dedication as "a note prefixed to a literary, artistic, or musical composition dedicating it to someone in token of affection or esteem."

"Token of affection or esteem" is hardly adequate for the dedications of this book.

This book is dedicated to the love of my life, my friend, and my hero—my wife, Pamela. We had a storybook romance that culminated with a wedding six months after our first date. People thought we were crazy to become engaged so soon, let alone be married, but we knew we were meant for each other. We have shared over thirty years of love, happiness, laughs, and adventure.

That life together began on the beautiful sand dunes in Pajaro Dunes, California. Overlooking the Pacific Ocean, watching the birds and seals and other animals, and gazing across an endless horizon gave us the impression that our life would be peaceful with only that horizon to chase.

Life has also included the ups and downs that people experience. Those good times and the tough times taught us a lot about life. But nothing could have prepared us for the portion of our journey that we are now living together.

My love has been by my side from the very first day this portion of our journey began. She was the link to our children. She was there for every doctor visit, every day in the hospital, and every visit to the pharmacy. She has been my chauffeur, my home care nurse, my emotional therapist, my physical therapist, my caregiver, and my advocate. She is the glue that kept our family together through the darkest days of our ordeal.

It is not an exaggeration for me to say that she saved my life. At several points in my treatment, she demonstrated that she knew me better than anyone else. She was an integral part of my professional team. She was indispensable in evaluating me and my condition as we made decisions every step of the way. I should say that I have recently learned that it was not "we" that made the decisions; with the advice of others, Pamela made most of the critical decisions.

Pamela was always with me—always in my heart even when I was not present mentally. She gave me hope with her voice, her constant reassurance, through tears, that I would survive. Her serene, ever-present smile brought warmth when I was cold, conditioned the air when I was warm, and filled every hospital room with light. I always knew she was there even though she did not know that I was aware of her presence.

I am forever indebted to her in so many ways. I owe her my life. These mere words cannot adequately express the way I feel.

I express my honor to have as my children two of the finest young adults I have ever known. Gerald and Jennifer, our now twenty-six-year-old twins, handled the news of my diagnosis with maturity and with commitment that I would be well. They were with me always.

As you raise your children, you often ask yourself whether you are doing a good job. As we say, the proof is in the pudding, and we cooked two good ones. In unexpected and remarkable moves, Gerald postponed the start of his career and Jennifer delayed graduate school to be there for me and for us. Each one moved back home for six-month stints to be with Pamela and help us through my illness.

They are remarkable young people, and if our future depends on people like them, I am confident we are in good hands.

Finally, I cannot express in words the feelings I have for a true angel, Andrew Wein. He saved my life and my family. I owe him more than any human being could ever give to another—the debt of life. He has made it clear to me that my survival is payment enough. And I pay equal tribute to his late wife, Sherry, and their son, Alexander, who are an integral part of this story as well.

**To Pamela, Gerald, Jennifer, and Andrew,
I dedicate this book—and I dedicate the rest of my life.**

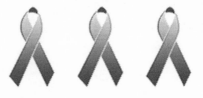

# CONTENTS

# ACKNOWLEDGMENTS

There are many people I have to thank for their help on this book. Those who played a key role are divided into three teams: my personal team, my professional team, and my health care team.

My personal team includes my family and friends, who have been a tremendous part of my support system, including my brothers, Mark and his wife, Carolyn, along with my other brother Lee and his wife, Wanda. Pamela's brother Kevin and his wife, Linda, were keys to our support and we always knew that Pamela's mother, Jan and her husband, Joe as well as Pamela's father Bill and his wife, Margaret were a part of our team as well.

I have great lifetime friends, but none greater than Karen Storey and Steve Tedesco. Karen managed a massive e-mail network, was a counselor to us, and flew to see us in Los Angeles at the drop of a hat whenever we needed anything. As a friend since kindergarten, Steve has been there for most of my life. He was as solid as a rock during this ordeal, handled many things for us, and gave me advice whenever I needed it—whether I asked for it or not. Their son, Sam, provided the comic relief we needed at just the right times.

Other friends were a big part of my personal team and their names are sprinkled throughout this book as I make specific reference to their contributions.

My professional team was led by my employer, the Los Angeles Area Chamber of Commerce. The chamber has been extremely supportive throughout, and for that I will forever be indebted. They gave me the opportunity to work while in treatment and recovery. They serve as a role model for how employers should treat people with serious illnesses. Beyond the chamber's volunteer leadership, board chairs Patty DeDominic, Charlie Woo, George Kieffer, Chris Martin, Dave Nichols, and David Fleming; the board of directors; the staff; and particularly Marlee Miller and David Eads displayed an unmatched loyalty, work ethic, professionalism, and level of support that kept the organization moving forward. I appreciate their support and honor their contributions. I also continued to rely on the support of chamber leaders from Sacramento including Raymond Nelson, one of my mentors, as well as others mentioned later in the book.

My health care team included hundreds of professionals who, at one time or another, were involved in my care. The principal members are listed here. I apologize, in advance, to any I have inadvertently omitted. Dr. Robert Watkins, MD, my orthopedic surgeon, first discovered the cancer. The University of Southern California team was headed by Dr. Aziz Khan, MD, (who diagnosed my leukemia) and included Dr. Daniel Douer, MD (hematology); Dr. Tony Talebi, MD (hematology/oncology); Dr. Robert Hagen, MD; and Dr. Gary Lieskovsky, MD (USC urologist). My nursing team at USC included Elizabeth Perez, Pat Ficzycz, Lisa Johnston, Justine Bo, Shane Kline, Tanya Price, Rose Balmaceda, Susan Wu, Teresa Lam, Maria Saigon, Connie Khatib, Susan Wu, Teresa Lam, Corazon Ferrer, and a wonderful transport guy—Andre Gonzales.

The City of Hope Team was led by Dr. Anthony Stein, MD, my principal physician and hematologist who managed my radiation treatments, transplant, and follow-up care at the City of Hope, and other members of his team included Dr. Pablo Parker, MD, and Dr. David Snyder, MD, (hematology); Dr. Geneisa Mahalingham, MD (cardiology); and Dr. Harry Openshaw, MD (neurologist); and Lynne Bonner, N.P., and nurses Jean Blalock, Kathy Neves, Debbie Vasquez, Mei Chung, Allison Sano, and Carol Schroeder.

Other LA doctors included Dr. Donald Norquist, MD, (orthopedic surgeon) and Dr. David Cannom, MD (cardiologist).

The team at Stanford is my active team now and is led by Dr. Robert Negrin, MD, (hematology/oncology) and included Drs. Sally Arai, MD, Keith Goldstein, MD, Judith Shizuru, MD, Gina LaPorte, MD, Gary Lowsky, MD, Michael Craig, MD, and Sam Mazj, MD, (hematology/oncology); Dr. Amin Al-Ahmad, MD, (cardiology); Dr. William Maloney, MD, (orthopedics); Dr. Tracey McLaughlin, MD, (endocrinology); Dr. Artis Montague, MD, (ophthalmology); Dr. Christopher Ta, MD, (ophthalmology); Dr. Ted Cooper, MD, (opthamology); Dr. Darius Moshfeghi, MD, (opthamology); Dr. Stephen Fischer, (anesthesia); Dr. Joseph Seppi Lin, MD, (pulmonology); Dr. John Adler, MD, (neurosurgery); Dr. Randall Vagelos, MD, (cardiology); Dr. Nikolas Blevins, MD, (otolaryngology); Dr. Andrea Natale, MD, of the Cleveland Clinic (a nationally known cardiologist who co-performed my atrial fibrillation ablation); and Joseph A. Ferrito, Au D. (audiology). The nursing staff at Stanford included Holly Sarocco, Judy Berry Price, Tina Jolly-Schmidt, Irish Jackman, Evelyn Barte, Iris Parris, Terry Langeman, Sandi Langeman, Sara Carney, Donna Clem, Lorna Arachea, Helen Benedetti, Donna Edwards, Colleen Carnathon, Laila Craveiro,

Laura DeBenning, Nimfa Fajardo, Trisha Jenkins, Gayla Knight, Anne Jacobs, Janet Metcalfe, Sherry Moore, Norine Mugler, Irene Page, Charize Paular, Stephanie Rocha, Joyce Sagun, Sara Strike, Yanli Wang, and Tsegreda Wubea. Support staff included Nirmala Singh, Arnel Solon, Malinda Law, Maggie Clark, Ellen Smiley, and Torey Benoit. I also would like to extend my appreciation to Grace Liu (physical therapy), and a very special man, Claro Calangi, who was always there to support me whether in transportation or any other special needs.

The team at Stanford also includes my friend, the president of the hospital, Martha Marsh. I am also indebted to Stanford's patient services group including Barbara Ralston and Judy Kaufman, who looked after me and solved many problems. In addition, I give special thanks to three extremely talented nurse practitioners, Lisa Mark (USC), Karen Harway (Stanford), and Ami Lombardi (Stanford), and to Lenny Navarro (a physician's assistant at Stanford).

Although there are far too many more to mention, I extend my thanks to the nurses at the above and other facilities who held my hand and heart during the long days and lonely nights. Indeed, some of the greatest nurses are those who know when to simply hold your hand and open their heart.

Some of the biggest heroes will never be on the front page of any newspaper, but they are true heroes in this fight. Finally, I offer my appreciation and thanks to other heroes in the war against cancer:

- To my fellow cancer patients, both those who have sacrificed and those who are survivors, who have helped the medical community learn important lessons and make astounding lifesaving breakthroughs

- To the doctors, researchers, medical professionals, and pharmaceutical companies who bring new technology, treatment, and medications to alleviate our pain and cure our illnesses

- To caregivers everywhere who put their lives on hold for months and years to provide the loving attention we need in difficult circumstances

- To families who suffer as much as we do and stay by our sides

- To the medical professionals and technicians who draw our blood and administer tests to monitor our progress

- And, to the nurses who are always by our side, at all hours of the day, providing the emotional support and expert medical advice we need

Without all of you, this journey would have been far different. On behalf of all of us, I extend to you our undying love and appreciation.

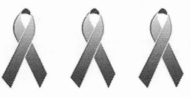

# WELCOME

Welcome.

My name is Rusty Hammer, and I have a rare form of a blood-related cancer. It is so rare that only one hundred cases like it are diagnosed in the United States each year. But I will tell you my story later.

What kind of cancer do you have?

I don't mean to scare you, but through my ordeal, I have learned that we all have potential cancer cells. The best way to think of it is that cancer cells are "good cells gone bad." Many of you don't have enough bad cells to form into active cancers, or you have an immune system that fights off cancers and other diseases.

By the summer of 2003, my immune system was not strong enough to fight the bad cells, and I developed cancer.

Throughout my treatment and recovery, which I now know will last a lifetime in many respects, my thoughts often shifted to what would happen if I did not have a good outcome. What would I leave my children? What would I leave as a legacy?

Responding to this I also give you a glimpse not only into my experience, but into my hopes and the life lessons we should all learn, which came to me clearly during some of the darkest days.

Before I approach the most important issues about what I learned and what I hope others can learn from me, I am going to take you through my experiences with leukemia. I have gone into detail about the trials of surviving the disease and the complications I faced, not to get sympathy or to exaggerate the challenges I have faced, but to give you a firsthand experience of not only what I went through but what I had to do to survive.

I have sprinkled my words with those from musicians, notable people, and other sources. Likewise I have turned to others who have traveled this road as I have, from patients to loved ones and caregivers. Their words convey messages that I could not express adequately myself.

I have been told by many people that the courage, tenacity, and will to live that I have displayed throughout this difficult journey have been an inspiration to others. I never meant this to be. I never meant to teach anything to anyone—just to survive to live another day.

Blood cancer is a deadly group of diseases that will claim over 55,000 lives this year. One person is diagnosed with a blood cancer every five minutes; one person dies every ten minutes; in total, over half a million people will die from cancer this year. But we can do something to reduce these numbers, to give people like me a second chance at life. You will learn more about that in this book as well.

I hope you will find value in learning about mine and my family's journey and that if you or your loved ones must face a major illness you will find kernels of wisdom and ideas in this book that will help you.

Please remember that I am not a doctor and am not giving any medical advice. You should always consult your doctor or other medical professionals and should not rely on anything that is contained in this book. I have tried to put in layman's terms what I have learned and, while physicians and health professionals may quibble with how I have explained some concepts, I have explained them in the best way I know how.

# INTRODUCTION

Cancer.

The C word.

It is a word that strikes fear in the hearts and minds of people whose lives are touched by it.

For me it was just a word until one fateful day that you will learn about as I share my experiences with you.

The reality of being diagnosed with cancer is something that you cannot understand until it happens to you. You can sympathize. You can empathize. You can feel sorry. But you cannot know how it feels until it happens to you. Nor can you understand how the treatments and side effects impact your life. But I have endeavored to bring to you as much reality as I can in this book as I have recounted my memories and descriptions of my experiences from diagnosis through today.

If this were just a memoir about my journey through cancer it might be interesting enough, but there are other memoirs you could read that would be equally interesting. That is why I decided to go several steps further and discuss how patients can better deal with a cancer diagnosis and how the medical community can better serve patients confronted with these dreaded diseases. And finally I have added some life lessons that I learned and wanted to impart to my wife, my children, and others.

I could not have survived my battle to this point without the help of many heroes along the way. Some of these heroes did their work before we were around. Some do their work today.

Many people wear these now familiar cancer ribbons designed to honor and pay tribute to those have lost or those who are engaged in the fight against cancer. Still others wear cancer bracelets popularized by Lance Armstrong, while others prefer to fight in private. However they choose to honor cancer's victims, these heroes deserve our recognition and our appreciation.

*Wind Beneath My Wings[1]*

Did you ever know that you're my hero?
… for you are the wind beneath my wings.
—Bette Midler

These words from Bette Midler ring so true, for the heroes in our lives give us the lift and the inspiration to be more than we think we can be on our own.

I would be nowhere in my fight against cancer today without the many heroes who have fought the fight before me. This book is as much about them as it is about me. Yet it is also written for those of you who will fight it in the months and years ahead; I want to arm you with the tools that will help you fight it.

I had my heroes in my battle—Vicki and Brian who have survived transplants for five and ten years, respectively. They went through similar treatments to mine and had different outcomes

---

1    http://www.azlyrics.com/lyrics/bettemidler/windbeneathmywings.html

and side effects. That is why I learned so much from each of them. They gave me the courage to move forward, one step at a time—one day at a time. They urged me on during the hardest of days. If there is anything that I can give you, it is this same determination to survive with courage and determination that they gave me.

Other heroes I focus on are those who have toiled in the laboratories, educational institutions, hospitals, and homes in the fight against cancer. The battle has been waged by these warriors for most of a century. It is one that is far from over and has already claimed too many victims. Unfortunately, it will claim far too many lives before the war can be won; indeed we may never be able to claim victory.

Recent strides in technology and knowledge have given health care providers the weapons to win battles they would have lost only decades or years earlier. In the case of leukemia, bone marrow transplants are once such weapon. Before they became a reality, though, doctors tried to save patients using the best protocols they had available—protocols that were unfortunately not enough to save hundreds of thousands. One such person, who I never met, was barely a teenager when he was diagnosed with a virulent form of leukemia that took his life a few short months later. His name was Jerry Richardson, and he would have been my brother-in-law.

People don't set out to be heroes. They are called. They may be called in an emergency. They may be called by an internal or religious passion. Similarly, people do not seek to be called by cancer.

> I think a hero is an ordinary individual
> who finds strength to persevere and endure
> in spite of overwhelming obstacles.
> —Christopher Reeve[2]

---

2    www.quotationspage.com.quote/34109.html

But when cancer calls it does so for a reason—just like every other calling that has its purpose. Cancer is nondiscriminatory. It calls the strongest and the weakest among us. It calls the most prepared and the least prepared. It calls the richest and the poorest. It calls the good people and those who do not practice goodness. People can do all of the right things in their treatment and lose the battle, and they can do all of the wrong things and win the battle. Those affected by the calling of cancer have no choice whether to answer the call. They must answer it in the best way they can. They will choose how to answer the call, not whether to answer it. Even if they give up, that, in itself, is an answer to the call; unfortunately, it is an answer that usually has dire consequences. Giving up is, in the worst of cases, a regrettable answer.

During my illness, former congressman, cabinet secretary, presidential candidate, and NFL quarterback Jack Kemp sent me a note along with the following quote:

> Never give in. Never, never, never, never, never!
> Never yield in any way, great or small.
> —Sir Winston Churchill[3]

People called by cancer do not know why they are so called. Only time, and how they handle that time, will determine how they answer the call.

I have no idea why I was chosen to take this journey down the cancer road. I can only hope that I was called because there is some good that will come of it, that I will find some positive contribution

---

3    Speech delivered in 1941 at the Harrow School

to make to those who will follow me down this road. Perhaps what I can give through this book is the first reason I received the calling.

As you will come to understand when you finish this book, there is probably no way this work should have been completed. I have been told so by most of my doctors. From developing a rare form of cancer to encountering what is an astounding list of complications impacting nearly every system of my body to facing emotional crises, my survival has been quite astonishing. Several health care providers have told me that I have been among the most complex cases they have ever seen. Beyond that, completing the book in such a short time period with the disabling list of issues I am dealing with has been difficult. But whatever the reasons, I have survived. I have summoned whatever is within me to get to this point and to be able to tell my story.

I hope that this will not be the last of my writing efforts. I encourage you to share with me your thoughts, ideas, and suggestions based on what you learn from this book. If you have ideas you would like to add to the list of suggestions, thoughts you would like to share with future readers, issues you would like me to write about, or other comments, please e-mail me at:

rusty@rustyhammer.com.

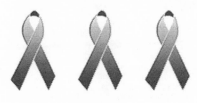

# PART I

# MY JOURNEY

# Chapter 1

# My Life Before Cancer

Our answer is the world's hope; it is to rely on
Youth—not a time of life but a state of mind, a temper of
the will, a quality of the imagination, a predominance of courage
over timidity, and the appetite of adventure over the love of ease.
—Robert F. Kennedy[4]

Senator Kennedy's words defined much of my life and have been a great source of inspiration in my work. As you learn about my life, you will find that Robert Kennedy is one of my heroes. I discovered these words as I became a teenager. In the pages that follow, you will see how profoundly they impacted me as I took on a life dedicated to community service and political activism at an early age.

This journey is about more than my travel through cancer because that journey must be placed in the context of my life experiences. The way I have responded to my call to cancer is, in many ways, the result of what I have learned and what I have experienced

---

4    Robert F. Kennedy, *To Seek a Newer World* (New York: Doubleday & Company, Inc., 1967), 232

over the past fifty-four years. And my resolve to recover and fight this dreaded disease is also influenced by those experiences.

The challenge that I faced, beginning in the summer of 2003, would be a steep hill to climb—steeper than any I could have imagined. But I have never taken the easy way out. My life has been defined by taking on tough challenges.

My story began over fifty years ago in Orleans, France, where I was born, in 1953, the second of three sons of Sidney and Birdie Hammer. My older brother, Mark, had been born three years earlier in Connecticut. My dad was in the army, and we just happened to be in France when the magic moment arrived for me.

My story almost ended quickly. I guess it was the beginning of my health problems, although no one could have predicted the direction they have taken.

My umbilical cord unraveled at birth, and I began to lose copious amounts of blood. The doctors began screaming that, unless transfusions were administered immediately, I would die. There was not enough time to do accurate blood typing and cross matching. They would have to make do with whatever blood was available. I received blood from nurses, doctors, soldiers, and officers. I survived my first challenge, and the transfusion scars remain like badges of courage on my ankles to this day. But those transfusions would hang over me during my cancer battle.

🎗 🎗 🎗

We settled in Virginia where my dad was stationed at Fort Belvoir. For the first five years of my life, I had an unremarkable childhood—snowboarding down the hills before it was the popular Olympic sport it is today, playing in the nearby schoolyard, and going to the army base regularly. In 1958, my second brother, Lee, was born, and my dad retired from the Army Corps of Engineers.

My mom and dad decided that they would pick up stakes and move to California as they had some army friends there, and California presented a great opportunity in the late '50s. We moved, first to the Monterey area near Fort Ord, but Seaside, California, did not suit my mother, so we picked up stakes and moved in with friends in San Jose. After a few months, they bought their first home in Campbell, California. Little did we know how the selection of the location of our home would influence my future.

I had a normal childhood: scouts, little league, good schools, and wonderful friends, many of whom are friends to this day. I received my Bar Mitzvah and also received the highest honor given by the Boy Scouts to Jewish scouts. I progressed to be a Life Scout (one merit badge short of Eagle). The lessons of being trustworthy, loyal, helpful, friendly, courteous, kind, obedient, cheerful, thrifty, brave, clean, and reverent defined my life.

But I am a bit ahead of myself.

I was anything but an athlete as a youngster. Sports did not interest me much; I was the studious one in the family. By the time I hit middle school, my teacher, Mrs. Conant, detected in me an interest in and aptitude for government and politics. It was 1964 (I was eleven years old), the year that Senator Barry Goldwater faced President Lyndon Johnson in Johnson's bid for his first full term as president. I was not much of a republican, so Mrs. Conant assigned me to be the floor manager representing President Johnson at a political convention that was held at our school. I went to Johnson's campaign headquarters regularly and really took to politics. I did so well that Mrs. Conant arranged for me an opportunity to serve as a page boy (they called them "boys" in those days) in the state legislature in Sacramento. It only magnified my interest in politics.

While in Sacramento, I ran errands for legislators, answered simple letters, sat in on meetings, and met people who would dominate California politics for the next forty years—people who remain friends today—from governors to legislators and mayors. I became involved in many political campaigns as a teenager and found any reason I could to be around political events from fund-raisers to county fairs. I recited the pledge of allegiance at political dinners and became known all around the county in political circles.

I got involved in every campaign I could. From stuffing envelopes to making calls, walking precincts, and miscellaneous tasks, I learned the political game from inside out. I loved it!

Once I reached high school, I was involved in student government and had the opportunity to work closely on Senator Robert Kennedy's campaign for president. I served as the chair of California High School Students for Kennedy and had the rare and humbling opportunity to meet Senator Kennedy in his hotel room during the last week of his life. It was one of the highlights of my life.

But that spark was extinguished with an assassin's bullet, which brought me to the realization that working to change things on the local level would be the best avenue for my energy. So I turned away from partisan politics and began to become involved in my community of Campbell. It was a small enough city that it afforded me the opportunity to make a difference. If we had moved to a big city years earlier, my options would have been different; this was perfect for me.

I worked on community projects. I became acquainted with community leaders and even applied for a seat on the planning commission but was turned down.

By this point, I was involved in student government in my high school and began to network with other student leaders. We began to talk about the need to involve young people in local government and we convinced the city council that young people were an important part of the community and that our input on issues impacting youth could help the city. Based on that advocacy, the city council formed the first youth advisory commission in the state of California, which I chaired when I was fifteen years of age. Comprised exclusively of young people, the commission was on the same level as all other city commissions (the planning commission, parks commission, etc.) and advised the city council on a variety of matters impacting young people, from recreation programs and crime to high school closures and parks issues.

I became intimately involved in community issues, and, when the voting age was lowered to eighteen in 1971, I decided to run for the city council against a sixteen-year incumbent. It was not for the lark of it; this individual and I had fundamental disagreements about the direction of the city, and I believed that the council needed a new voice. I was taking this very seriously; I planned to win. Nobody thought I could win, but they treated me with respect. How could an eighteen-year-old win election to the city council? Preposterous!

I walked every neighborhood, knocked on nearly 90 percent of the doors in the city, and, improbably, was elected—at that time the youngest elected official in U.S. history. The morning after the election, cameras and reporters flooded Campbell to report the news; even a reporter representing the *London Times* was there. Three years later, I became mayor, at the age of twenty-one, the youngest mayor in U.S. history, earning me a feature on ABC's *AM America* (now called *Good Morning America*).

This would be my first real lesson that commitment and perseverance brings huge rewards. It is a lesson that I hope I would pass on to my children throughout their lives.

Once I became mayor, I repaid Mrs. Conant for introducing me to politics by appointing her to a city commission, and I later helped her get elected to the city council in her own right.

The next twelve years were a whirlwind. I participated in everything I could in local and regional government. At one time or another, I served on over fifty committees throughout the San Francisco Bay area working on issues impacting youth, transportation, seniors, health care, poverty—you name it. If there was a need, I was there. I was involved in The League of California Cities and the National League of Cities. I spoke at conferences around the state and nation. During this time, I held two jobs, graduated from the Santa Clara University with an undergraduate degree in political science, and obtained a master's degree in public administration. It was 1975. I get tired now just thinking about how busy I was!

At that point in my life, I aspired to become involved professionally in city administration, perhaps as a city manager. But finding a job was difficult because no city would hire me given that I was on the council in another city. I was not interested in giving up my political career at that time. As a result, I decided to work as a political and public relations consultant for a few years until I could sort out my goals more clearly.

Looking back on it, those young adult years laid the foundation for how I would approach my life for the next thirty. To say that I attended many events and sat on many committees is an understatement. I was totally consumed by the political life. Imagine attending city council meetings and committee meetings every week. Meetings would often last until after midnight, often several nights a week. I was always available for my constituents in person or by telephone. Phone calls came 24/7 about every subject you could imagine.

I received calls about barking dogs and garbage pickups. I rode on shifts with police officers and fire fighters. I worked with street repair and vehicle repair crews so that I could understand exactly what they did.

I was everywhere, all the time. Because I was so extensively covered in the media due to my age, people would just walk up to me in the store or on the street. This pace brought me the burdens of pneumonia and mononucleosis, which tried to slow me down. But I seldom paid attention to the warnings—I was on the fast track doing important things. The challenge ahead was to keep my political career moving forward, earn a living, and start a family.

I had great success. Along with a coalition on the council, we built needed parks and neighborhood facilities, built up fiscal reserves, established recreation programs and a downtown redevelopment program, saved a closing high school and converted it into a community center, and accomplished many other things I took great pride in. An interesting coincidence is that Steve Tedesco, my great friend, was president of the school board, and it was the two of us who worked together to make sure that the city of Campbell and the school district worked together to allow the high school to be saved as a community center. This back story is one that few people, to this day, are aware of.

The love of my life entered my world in early 1976. Pamela brought brightness, warmth, compassion, intelligence, humor, and balance to my life. After a short courtship, we married in the summer of 1976. Pamela's mother, Jan, introduced us. Jan and I had been working on improving access to the disabled community when she invited me over to dinner to meet her new husband, Joe. I agreed and called for directions a few days before the dinner. At that point I knew she was up to something when she said, "Now, you wouldn't mind if my daughter joined us, would you?" I had no choice.

Pamela and I didn't see each other for months due to my busy travel schedule (and because I was rather shy), but, once we started dating, the attraction was immediately clear, and we were married within six months. It was a whirlwind that has continued for over thirty years.

For the next two years, I pursued my consulting business and political career, and Pamela worked in the medical field. We struggled financially but made it through. We were able to buy our first home the year we were married just as the housing market took off in California. By 1978, I was being urged to run for higher political office and that year decided that I would run for the state legislature. It was a hard-fought campaign against an entrenched incumbent, but it left a bitter taste in my mouth because I did not receive the support from party leaders I had expected. As a result, the money to run an effective campaign was not available and, unfortunately,

I fell just short of being elected. It changed our lives forever, but in more positive ways as we would soon learn.

When you think you will travel one road—the political one—and lose an election, you are devastated and think your life is over, and I believed that to be the case. For several months, I felt that my life was over. But Pamela and I were young and just married, and before long we were back to approaching life with zeal.

The first change I made was to decide to pursue a career in the private sector rather than in politics. Henceforth, politics would be an avocation rather than a career. I joined a local engineering firm, working in public and investor relations. As usual, I bit off more than I could chew. When something needed to be done, mine was the first hand in the air. Promotions came rapidly as I took on assignments for which I had few qualifications. But I learned on the fly and bulldozed my way to accomplishment and success.

By two years later, when the legislative position was once again up for grabs, I had taken a hard look at the results of the previous campaign and realized that I had done all that I could have in the race and had lost not because of a lack of effort but because the party had not supported me adequately. I figured that, if they did not care, there was no reason for me to put myself out again and take the same risk. So I decided to sit it out. And sure enough, the party leaders sat the race out again for the next candidate.

By early 1980, Pamela and I began to seriously discuss having a family. We both wanted children and, now that the political bug had been extinguished and I was somewhat ensconced in the private sector, it was a good time to begin. Six months after we learned Pamela was pregnant, we were at her doctor's office, and, as the nurse was listening to the heartbeat, she said, "I am not sure, but I either hear an echo or two heartbeats." The next day an ultrasound confirmed that we were having twins.

We were numb. We would get the two children we wanted—but all at once? We could never do things the easy way. For the next three months, we were the center of attention as city hall, friends, and the office held polls: would we have two boys? Two girls? One of each? As for names, they played on my name: Sledge Hammer, Jack Hammer, Claw Hammer, you name it—they came up with it.

After Gerald and Jennifer were born, the world did not stop, much less slow down. I continued to receive promotions at Quadrex Corporation, under the guidance of one of my lifetime mentors, our chairman, Sherman Naymark, one of the classiest, most intelligent men I have ever had the honor to know. Sherman hired me at the urging of his son, Ron, and gave me the unique opportunity to work in all areas of corporate management, as a vice president of human resources, chief financial officer, president of an operating business unit, and president of our international subsidiary. It was a unique experience because I was one of few nonengineering executives in an engineering company.

Sherman allowed me to take on assignments throughout the company and learn corporate management governance and principles from top to bottom. It was a unique experience. But it was more than that. I soaked up his every word, his every lesson, his every view and perspective. I learned from an exceptional man who had a distinct perspective on people, business, and management. The range of these experiences ultimately led me to serve as president and chief executive officer of the company and a member of the board of directors. What Sherman taught me about management, compassion, and the techniques of corporate governance molded my career for the last thirty years. It gave me an opportunity to do staff and operational management. I did mergers and acquisitions, finance, worked with Wall Street; you name it, I did it. I traveled the world extensively, racking up millions of air miles and frequent flyer points—so many that I lost most of them because I could never use them.

I worked like a madman. One year I was in Germany twelve times overseeing a subsidiary company that was in trouble. I remember another period when I spent two weeks in Japan, came home for one day to California, and flew to Germany for a week; then I was back in California for two days before leaving for ten days in Taiwan.

I kept an exhausting schedule, working twelve plus hours a day for six or seven days a week. I often did not know whether I was coming or going. Perhaps the worst example was one day when I came home at lunch to prepare to leave for Europe. The kids were less than a year old, and Pamela was sitting down in the family room, feet up on the cedar chest. She was not walking around; I was rushing like a madman. I was somewhat irritated that she was not helping until she told me that she had broken her ankle that morning in a restaurant parking lot. But I had no choice; I had to go. So we arranged a maid to help her out for the week I would be gone—and off I went.

I justified this workaholic pace out of the need to provide the best I could for my young and growing family. We needed the money. I needed the challenges; there was so much I wanted to accomplish. And despite the heavy work schedule, I kept myself in touch with the family and am proud that I never missed a birthday, anniversary, school play, or other important event. Somehow, through it all, I was able to coach Gerald's baseball and soccer teams and Jennifer's softball and soccer teams and serve as PTA president.

But I was simply justifying things as it took a toll on me and on our family. I was not home as much as I would have liked. Pamela took the lead role in raising our children. And to this day, I hope that the pace of my life did not wear down my immune system and lead to my leukemia, although doctors have reassured me that this is likely not the case.

By the time the kids were nine, the company was undergoing major changes, which required our relocation to Florida. Although we had been Californians our entire life, the opportunity to move to another part of the country seemed exciting. It would be a chance to learn about another area, experience new people, and have new adventures. We stayed in Florida for four years, during which time I became president and CEO of Quadrex Corporation. This period required an even greater amount of travel and time commitment. One evening I recall that I was conducting a board meeting on the telephone and, during the meeting, had an anxiety attack that felt much like a heart attack. I spent two days in the hospital, but of course I did not leave for the hospital until the board meeting had ended!

By early 1993, the company's future was in doubt due to decisions that had been made by the prior CEO. It was then that I took over the reigns. In late 1993, I presented a turnaround plan to the board that they did not accept because it focused more on our traditional businesses which, while lower-margin, were profitable nonetheless. Unfortunately, they were not the ones that created the "sizzle" and high stock prices demanded by Wall Street. I was much more interested in building the business for the long term rather than for short term profits. Based on that disagreement over the strategic direction of the company, I resigned. I suppose the vindication of my recommendations was that the company filed Chapter 11 bankruptcy and was sold off in pieces within a year.

While all of this was occurring, I was looking after my mother who had become seriously ill. She and my dad had talked about moving to Florida to be with us and make a new life there, and after Mom had undergone repeated medical treatment in California, we had brought my parents to Florida. There she received more treatments, which unfortunately were not successful.

We then decided to return to California.

We stayed in Florida for about nine months after I left Quadrex while I worked as a financial consultant for a company in New Jersey that produced Nintendo game platforms. Basically I served as the company's outsourced Chief Financial Officer and a board member. It was a fun opportunity because it was my first opportunity to work with a consumer goods company, and it was a turnaround as well. But after nine months, I was given an opportunity to return to California.

California was always our home, and once I let people know that I wanted to return, I'd known it would just be a matter of time before the right opportunity would open up for me. In mid-1994, I received a call from a recruiter about an opportunity to become the Sacramento Metropolitan Chamber of Commerce's president and chief executive officer. I suppose I was on the list because of my reputation as an executive and my political expertise. It was an opportunity for me to become reengaged in public policy and political issues that launched my career. It was a high profile job in the state capitol and an opportunity to move in a new direction. On the other hand, the organization was a nonprofit, so I would always need to be raising money. But the organization was one hundred years old, and it had financial reserves on its balance sheet so that should not be a concern. After looking at its financial statements and meeting with its executive committee and officers those concerns were allayed. They made an offer and I accepted.

Unfortunately, a week after I arrived I would learn that things are not always as they appear on paper. The biggest part of the challenge was that it was a turnaround. The chamber was technically bankrupt when I arrived, although neither the board nor I knew it. It spent money it did not have. Stale checks were stuffed in drawers, and payables were not accounted for. The chamber was disorganized and lacked focus. It had lost its place as the premiere business organization in the region.

My mission was to turn it around and fix it. I jumped right into the challenge. It was right up my sleeve. The chamber would be the proud and great organization it once was. I thought it would take five years.

We took bold steps, made many changes, developed a strategic plan, re-staffed the organization, entered new business areas, and started new events—all directed at restoring this one-hundred-year-old organization to prominence and financial stability. The plan worked, and today the chamber is all that we thought it would become.

The biggest gamble I took was in my first full year. That year we would celebrate our one hundredth anniversary, and I thought we needed to develop a major event to commemorate it. Without spending a lot of space here explaining it, I conceived of an event we called Perspectives, a daylong speakers' program that brought national and international speakers to discuss issues of importance to the country and the world. Over the years, speakers have included former U.S. presidents George H. W. Bush, and Gerald Ford, General Colin Powell, British prime minister Margaret Thatcher, California governor Arnold Schwarzenegger (before he was governor), British prime minister John Major, New York governor Mario Cuomo, John Glenn, Israeli prime minister Benjamin Netanyahu, Israeli prime minister Shimon Peres, Canadian prime minister Brian Mulroney, and many others. Speakers were not only political; they included former NFL quarterback Terry Bradshaw, comedian Rich Little, Mt. Everest climber and motivational speaker Dr. Beck Weathers, and many more. Perspectives became an annual event.

The year we began the program we had no money to pay the speakers, so I turned to one of the chamber's board members and a great friend, who ultimately was elected to the chamber chairmanship and the Sacramento County Board of Supervisors, Susan Peters and her late husband Peter McCuen who loaned us the money for a down payment on the speaker fees. Fortunately, we nearly broke even and made up the small loss in the second year. Perspectives was the biggest (and best) financial and programmatic risk in the organization's history. Hosting the program that first year was exactly the kind of risk that executives take when they are faced with all-or-nothing circumstances and they have the confidence in themselves, their strategy, and their staff to execute a plan. Today it is the largest moneymaker for the chamber and has saved the organization financially. Today the program has become by far the largest annual public affairs event in the Sacramento region and has restored the chamber's reputation as a leading forum for public and political affairs.

That, along with a long list of other initiatives, elevated the chamber to unequaled status in Sacramento. The turnaround was successful in just a few years. At one time we had to beg people to join the chamber board. In just a short few years business leaders competed to join the board. It was a dramatic turn of events in which I and the people who were a part of the team took great pride.

Unfortunately, I did not learn the lessons that my earlier life should have taught me. I jumped into a work-dominated life—being everywhere, doing everything. By this time, Gerald and Jennifer were in high school and becoming somewhat independent. Pamela was as well, as she became involved in her career in real estate. Sadly, we found that our four lives were beginning to move in somewhat different directions.

As we tried to do everything we could for our children, Pamela and I did not pay as much attention as we should have to each other. We let our health become less of a priority, didn't take enough time off, and saw stress take over our lives.

But I was successful. I was providing for my family. I was well respected in the community, and I was in the media constantly. I gave my family reasons to be proud of me. That was what I told myself they wanted. But I soon learned that no matter how well I did professionally or financially, if I was not there with my family nurturing my relationships with them, they would move forward on their own. The growing distance between us got serious until we decided to seek counseling and a realistic look at our future intervened and put us back on the right track after we had been together for twenty-five years. The love we shared for each other was too strong for us to give up.

It was the second time in my life that I learned that perseverance and never giving up hope pays huge rewards.

By 2001, after seven years in Sacramento, another intervening event fell into our lives that gave us an opportunity to redefine our future. I was heavily recruited to take over the Los Angeles Area Chamber of Commerce as its president and CEO. Think of it—the opportunity to be the leader of the business community of the country's second largest city, and it was another turnaround at that, only on a larger scale. All of us in the industry knew that the LA Chamber was a mess. It was on a downhill trajectory and likely headed for bankruptcy. Only a miracle would save it. I enjoyed my job in Sacramento and was secure enough to call it a career there in another ten years.

But LA? What a tremendous career opportunity! No respectable northern Californian would leave the calm, excellent climate and quality of life of the north for LA. I thought about it for a long time. I loved Sacramento. I loved the job. I loved the people. Pamela had a great career. I said no to three calls from LA.

But I just could not see myself giving up the ultimate career opportunity on the ultimate stage. That just was not in me. The fourth time the chamber called, I had dinner with one of their board members, George Kieffer, in Sacramento, for nearly four hours. We clicked on so many levels.

I reported for work in Los Angeles on November 5, 2001.

I was in Los Angeles in the dream job that I thought would define the later years of my career. The organization had lost more than a million dollars the year before I arrived and several millions in the years before. Membership has been on a ten-year downward trend. Its influence had been waning. But I could not have been more excited.

I was alone in an apartment for six months before Pamela was able to sell our house in Sacramento and move down to Los Angeles. It was a period of nonstop work for me.

The Chamber had seventy-five board members, and I insisted on meeting with each one of them. If you know Los Angeles, you realize how spread out the area is and how difficult that task was. Undaunted, I accomplished it. I went to nearly every social event I was invited to. I met with organizations and corporate leaders that were not represented on the board. I established relationships that would prove helpful in the months and years ahead. I met with members of Congress and the legislature who had become disaffected with the chamber. I attended city council meetings and met with anyone who would meet with me. My matrix of people, organizations, and businesses was full and complete, and I applied all of my energies to the tasks at hand.

The first year was difficult. I had to assess the tools I had available to me in the form of people assets. Who were the performers? Who could we do without? What were the near term priorities? What could we afford? What should our one year, two year, and three year business plans look like? What about a five year strategic plan? Decisions had to be made daily as the chamber was bleeding cash as it had been for years.

Fortunately, one of my strengths is in the area of business turn-arounds, and the plan I put together worked. By the end of the first year, we had turned things around. Profitability returned. Membership was on a growth curve. Political support returned.

The board could not have been more pleased. I was at the top of my game and developing a new strategic plan that would assure our growth for the coming five years. Nothing could stop us.

Once Pamela moved down and we'd settled in the most beautiful home we had ever owned, we began living a life of culture, diversity, excitement, and personal accomplishment that was truly a whirlwind. We were around fun people—those who cared little about our bloodline and more about what we could do. One thing I discovered about LA is that it surely is a place where people look to you to make promises and deliver, and if you do, you are accepted. It was what I excelled at.

From a business standpoint, the turnaround I promised the LA chamber was well underway. Pamela and I had placed concrete in the footsteps of our relationship. I was learning to balance my personal and professional life in a way I had never done before. The kids were in college and were close by—Gerald at UC Irvine and Jennifer at UCLA. Things could not have been better for us. Most of all, we were in control of our lives. We aspired to have control so that we could set our own destiny and, for the most part, we were successful. We were living good and productive lives. We had great kids, made a good living, mingled with wonderful people, and achieved major professional accomplishments. It seemed that we were destined to continue down that path.

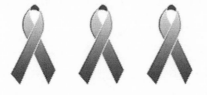

# CHAPTER 2

# THE NIGHTMARE BEGINS

Courage is being scared to death but saddling up anyway.

—John Wayne[5]

A few months before leaving for LA, Pamela and I had been in an automobile accident caused by a teenage driver in Sacramento. I'd had some back pain and was being seen by a doctor, but it seemed bearable. As the months went along the pain increased, and I had started seeing a doctor in Sacramento. There had been no conclusive results; I'd learned that it was probably just deep tissue injuries, so life went on. It was one random occurrence that, for some reason, would take us down a road that, for the first time in our lives, would spin us totally out of control.

In May, 2003, Pamela planned two surprise parties for my fiftieth birthday. One was at PacBell Park to watch the San Francisco Giants, my favorite baseball team. Over twenty people joined us that day; it was one of the best days of my life. The other was held in Los Angeles for the good friends we'd made there. As it would

---

5    www.quotationspage.com/quote/2111/html

turn out, these days would be the last real celebrations for years to come. There was no inclination, no warning that anything inside me was awry.

## Diagnosis

It was the spring of 2003. Things could not have been much better for the Hammer family. We were settled in Los Angeles, and I was having great success at work. Pamela and I were closer to each other than we had been in several years. Gerald and Jennifer were in their final years in college. A long-planned trip to Europe celebrating their graduation and fiftieth birthdays of several of our friends was set for the summer. Pamela was getting involved in a foundation that was working with improving opportunities for inner-city youth in LA.

I was feeling fine and had no symptoms of any illness. My blood tests, which were done as a part of my annual physical exams, were completely normal. Most people with cancer have abnormally high levels of white cells or other markers that give clues that something is amiss. But not so with me.

I was being seen by an orthopedic surgeon in Los Angeles for a continuing back problem resulting from the automobile accident. My doctor ordered tests to get a closer look at some inflammation that showed up on my lower back X-rays. He ordered a bone scan, a positron emission tomography (PET) scan, a magnetic resonance imaging (MRI), and a computed tomography (CT) scan.

If you have never had these tests, this explanation will help you understand what is involved:

Bone Scan:

A bone scan is a test that identifies bone growth or break-down. It is used to evaluate damage to the bones, detect cancer that has spread to the bones, and monitor conditions that can affect the bones (including infection and trauma). To conduct a scan, the patient receives an injection of a radioactive substance that is injected into a vein in the arm. Images are taken several hours later to show the presence of cancer, fracture, or an infection. Beyond the injection, and laying on a hard table for about an hour, it is a painless procedure.

PET Scan:

A PET scan (also usually combined with a CT scan), is also an invasive radioactive procedure. The patient is injected with a radioactive tracer that looks for and attaches to tumors that are fast growing and usually indicative of a malignancy. The substance is injected through an IV and circulates in the body for about an hour. The patient is then taken to the scanner, which is a long tube on a very hard table.

Depending on your size, there are literally only inches between you and the sides of the tube, and you are of course totally encased. You are in big trouble if you are claustro-phobic. One hospital gave me a dose of medication to put me at ease, but most of the time I did it without the aid of any medications.

Once you are inside the tube, the table moves ever so slowly from your head to your feet while you hold your hands and arms over and behind your head. It is a very uncomfortable position. You must hold that position and not move for an hour or more. It is an exhausting procedure.

## MRI:

An MRI scan can be invasive (using injected radioactive tracers) or noninvasive (without injection), but is not based on radiation as are bone scans and PET scans. Instead, it uses magnetic and radio wave technology to look at tissues in the body from all angles. The scanner is much like a PET scanner. The machine is just as small and claustrophobic. Unlike a PET scan, which is essentially silent, an MRI scan is extremely loud. The sound is caused by the banging together of the magnetic and radio waves. It is so loud that you must wear earplugs during the test.

## CT Scan:

A CT scan, known also as a CAT scan, also uses radioactive principles to look at tissues, organs, etc. It used to be that the scanners were also full body scanners, but recent advances have made them much smaller. Today, you seldom see a full body scanner. Instead, just a portion of the body is inserted in the machine, making it much less claustrophobic and inhibiting.

Before undergoing these scans, or any tests for that matter, you should ask a number of questions to satisfy yourself that the tests are necessary. Some that I would suggest are:

- What is the purpose of the test?
- Why do I need it?
- What other tests could uncover the same information?
- What happens if I don't have the test?
- What is the cost?
- Are there less expensive alternatives?
- Can the test give a false positive? How will we know?
- Is there any pain?
- Will you explain how the test is conducted?
- When will I get the results?
- Are there other tests needed to confirm the results?
- Will it be uncomfortable?
- What preparation must I do in advance?

In late May, the results were in from the tests on my back. Pamela and I went to see Dr. Watkins, certain that he would be recommending a surgical solution to address my back pain and just as certain that we would want to say no. My dad had been through several back surgeries and was never the same. I knew that I did not want to end up like he had—disabled and in constant pain.

Dr. Watkins came into the room, sat down, and opened my chart, obviously for the first time that day. Bob had become a good friend, having been referred to me by the owner of the Los Angeles Dodgers as he was the team physician as well. During visits, Bob and I would talk a lot about the business issues facing LA and politics. I always enjoyed my visits with him.

Not this time.

He turned as white as a ghost as he read the chart. After a few moments, he looked up and said, "Rusty, I don't know how to say this, but it looks like we need to forget about your back for a while … it appears that you have cancer."

I gripped Pamela's hand. One of us, perhaps both, started shaking in disbelief. I know for sure that we both were crying as Bob took us out of the room and to his private office. I know that Bob shared our emotions as well. His reaction was genuine, as was his high level of concern. He explained that the scans indicated that I had a spot on my prostate and in several other locations that the radiologist diagnosed as possibly being prostate cancer and that it appeared that the cancer has metastasized to several other places.

He told us that he'd had prostate cancer several years ago and that it had been treated by a doctor at the University of Southern California (USC). He immediately picked up the phone and made an appointment for us to see Dr. Gary Lieskovsky the next day. Bob assured me that, if caught early, my prognosis was excellent. With his assuring words, we went away scared but optimistic.

By ordering those tests, Dr. Watkins saved my life.

I remember going home that evening, and it was still light outside. We could not stay in the house, so we took one of our usual walks through San Marino and South Pasadena. I don't remember what we said to each other specifically; we cried a little. Mostly I remember that we were numb and kept asking each other what we would do.

I do not know today why we were chosen, nor does it matter. What really matters is what we did with our new life. The balance of our lives would be different, and my focus would be different.

You will have to pardon the analogy, but hearing you have cancer literally and figuratively scares you to death. You have two choices—you can either accept that you have a fate that may cause your premature death, or you can resolve to fight and defeat it. It takes courage to do the latter—as John Wayne says, to saddle up in the face of adversity. For those of you facing cancer, please know that it will take all of the courage and intensity you will be able to summon from within.

Nothing is more difficult to deal with than being diagnosed with a terminal illness. Years ago, the C word was almost certainly a death sentence. Although certain cancers are curable, and people are living longer with cancer, a cancer diagnosis still creates fear and uncertainty. Those of you who have recently been diagnosed are at the precipice of a long and uncertain journey; nevertheless, you need to muster all that is inside of you and move forward along your journey.

How does one cope with one's own mortality? We all know that we will die someday; when that day will come is one of the great mysteries of life. But when actually confronted with a diagnosis that you have a disease that may take your life sooner than you planned, the prospect of confronting that mystery becomes all too real.

Surviving cancer is a journey; there is really no specific day on which cancer begins. It is a marathon, not a sprint. I say there is no beginning because cancer, unlike breaking a bone, does not really begin on a specific day that we recognize. We don't know that we have it when it starts; we only know we have it when we are diagnosed. And that is where the journey begins—for the patient and for his or her family, friends, and loved ones.

Take it from me, that news can be devastating. When I was told, it was as though I had been hit in the stomach with a baseball bat. All of the wind was knocked out of me. Could I have given it to my kids? Did I inherit it? Am I going to die from it? When? There were so many questions and not enough answers.

And too often, a diagnosis comes too late. Fortunately for me, mine was early enough to give me reason to be hopeful.

The next day we were at the University of Southern California's Norris Cancer Center. Dr. Lieskovsky ordered some tests and gave me the usual examination, and we set an appointment for a week later. His initial conclusion was that he did not sense a prostate tumor based on the physical examination but that additional tests were needed.

The intervening days would comprise the longest week of our then twenty-seven years together. We cried out of uncertainty. We took long walks in the evening and discussed our fears about our children, the house, money, insurance benefits, and what my dear wife would do if things did not go well.

Were our papers in order? What about wills, advanced directives, taxes, and the myriad of other details? How would we face up to the challenges that were in store for us? Would I see our children marry and start families? Would there be grandchildren in our future, and would they ever sit on my lap or be caressed in my arms?

It was a scary time. We could focus on little else.

We read about prostate cancer on the Internet and in a *Newsweek* magazine, which just that week had a cover story on the topic. We talked to friends who had been through it. And we circled around as a family and with a few key friends who would become an integral part of our journey. I was ready for prostate cancer and had studied enough that I knew the direction I would go with my treatment. I was assured by many friends that prostate cancer had become one of the more curable cancers and that I should relax and be confident about the future.

I knew everything one could know about prostate cancer even before I knew I had it.

By the day of my next appointment, we were ready for the news. But the news was not what we expected. My prostate specific antigen (PSA) test was within the normal range, as was the free PSA test, which is a more detailed analysis. The prostate examination showed that my prostate, while enlarged, did not appear to have a tumor. In short, the likelihood that I had prostate cancer, much less the possibility that it had spread, was extremely low, and more tests were needed. Given that there was a spread of some type of cancer, we were all unsure of what these results meant.

It seemed hard to believe, but what might have been relief that I did not have prostate cancer strangely frightened us even more. We were back in no-man's-land because we did not know what we were dealing with. It was good news, but it was accompanied by a wave of uncertainty, because they were sure that I had cancer of some type.

At this point, Dr. Lieskovsky suggested that I see a radiologist who would take a biopsy to determine the type of cancer with which we were dealing.

Following the appointment, Pamela and I went back to my office. Now that we were back in the land of uncertainty, we decided it was time to begin to tell a few people that something was wrong. It would only be a matter of time before they figured it out anyway, so we felt an overwhelming need to share our feelings.

The first person we told was my coworker, Marlee Miller. She was more than a coworker; she was a friend and confidant whom I'd hired in Sacramento and recruited to LA. She would be with us every step of the way.

As it turned out, my LA mentor, George Kieffer, was in the office that day. George was more than a mentor. It was George who recruited me to LA with our shared vision about what we could accomplish together. We had shared political values. Our links to the Kennedy legacy were clearly related. We had similar views about the role the chamber should play in building the region. He was one of the most intelligent and brilliant leaders I have ever known. I would not have taken the job without him. He was a visionary and compassionate man. George did not know about the possibility of a cancer diagnosis, but when he walked into my office, Pamela completely lost her composure. At that point we shared our sad news with George.

George held her and reassured her that he and the Chamber would be by my side. He instantly became part of our support circle.

We spent some time at the office and then went home. After telling Pamela's family and my brothers, the most difficult call was to Steve and Karen, close friends for years—I'd known Steve since childhood. I was not able to get through more than a minute of the call before turning it over to Pamela, who was equally emotional.

Their first reaction was what we would have expected; they pledged to be right there with us every step of the way. Little did we know just how much that would mean over the next few years.

Subsequent calls were made to other friends, but we decided to keep the circle as small as possible. Without a firm diagnosis, the only thing we could tell them was that I was sick—probably with cancer—but there were too many questions we could not answer.

It may sound hard to believe, but for the first time I was thankful that my parents were no longer with us. I had been close to my parents and loved them very much, but the mere thought of having to having to tell them that I had cancer and might die would have been too much to bear. I have talked with many people who have told me that a parent's nightmare is to have a child pass away before them. In some strange way, their death was a blessing, for it saved me the most difficult conversation that I would ever have had.

We decided not tell the kids just yet. They would soon be graduating from college, and we did not want to distract them in their final weeks. We wanted them focused and happy during one of the most important times of their young lives. Their graduation would occur the following month and, by the coincidence of timing, their graduations were to occur on the same day, at the same time, at two different universities. We could wait that long. It would be selfish of me to invade their happiness.

When their special day came, we split up the graduation duties. I went to Gerald's at the University of California in Irvine and Pamela went to Jennifer's at UCLA. We watched them separately and welled up with pride simultaneously as our two young adults received their diplomas that licensed them to go out into the world and pursue their life ambitions.

We gathered for parties later in the evening with their groups of friends and families as if nothing was amiss. Everyone was happy all weekend as Pamela and I carried our hearts in our shoes. But we gutted it out, not wanting to spoil one of the best days of their lives.

After things settled down, we knew that the time had come to tell them that something was seriously wrong. We told them that we did not know much at that point but that I had something seriously worrisome going on with my health. We skirted around the C word, but they read our eyes, emotions, and body language. We told them that we did not know specifically what it was but would know soon after a planned biopsy and vacation. They were courageous, while shedding a few tears, and anxious, as we all were, to get some answers.

Now that we knew it was not prostate cancer, we had to get back to finding out what was wrong with me.

The tests showed that the largest of my tumors was located on my spine; it was unrelated to the back problems I was having as a result of the car accident. Dr. Lieskovsky referred us to Dr. Aziz Khan at USC who specialized in lymphoma, leukemia, and related cancers. We were not sure why we were being transitioned to a physician who specialized in these areas, but we didn't focus on it; we just wanted answers.

Dr. Khan recommended that I undergo a needle biopsy, in which a needle would be inserted into one of the tumors to get a sample of tissue. That would give them an opportunity to study the tissue and make a complete diagnosis. The biopsy was scheduled for a week later, which was early June, 2003.

That meant another week of uncertainty—of knowing that something was growing inside of me that could be shortening our life together.

The biopsy was a semi-surgical procedure. I was given a relaxing medication (Ativan—it's good stuff), and thirty minutes later the radiologists had their sample.

After a seemingly unending week of waiting, we were told that the results of the biopsy were, once again, inconclusive. They could not make a specific diagnosis. More delay. More uncertainty. More walks through the neighborhood in the twilight hours. More days at the office pretending nothing was wrong. More hiding the real truth from the kids. More nights crying ourselves to sleep.

Given the uncertainty, Dr. Khan told us that the only way to obtain a definitive diagnosis, upon which treatment could be based, was to conduct a full surgical biopsy. Such a procedure would be done by a thoracic surgeon. In the two-hour procedure, they would make several incisions in my back and collapse my lung in order to gain access to the principal tumor on my spine. It was a serious procedure. Penetrating and collapsing the lung would pose signifi-cant risk that would probably keep me hospitalized for a week.

As much as I did not want to go through the pain of this biopsy and the risk of surgery, we knew that we had no choice. The kids agreed. It was the only way to get a definitive answer. The biopsy was scheduled for late June.

I was admitted to the USC University Hospital in late June, and I went home on July 3. The surgery was relatively uneventful, although painful. The surgical team successfully obtained the sample, but a week later we received a call informing us that the initial results were, again, inconclusive and needed more study. Postsurgical pain was intense as they had had to cut through a significant number of nerves in my chest and back. Every move I made, every time Pamela touched me, every time my shirt moved aggravated those nerves and caused pain.

We were in the twilight zone. Everything was coming back inconclusive. Did we have the right doctors? Did they know what they were doing? How could things be so uncertain? Did we need to go elsewhere for answers?

In addition, we were preparing to leave on a long-planned vacation to Europe. How could we embark on such a long and joyous celebration with such uncertainty hanging over our heads? It would be an ambitious trip on barges and bicycles. I was in terrible pain from the surgery and feared that I would be miserable during the trip.

The doctors told us they were sure they could make a diagnosis, but they simply needed more time and had to involve other people in studying the tissues and developing a definitive diagnosis. They urged us to go to Europe and have a good time (right!) and told us we would know something when we returned home.

So we did. We really had no choice. It was the right decision. We would have been miserable at home if we had not taken the trip, and we needed something positive on which to focus. And, I needed to put on my game face and keep a stiff upper lip, if for no reason other than not to alarm our friends.

Additionally I learned an important lesson that I would apply throughout my treatment. Sometimes the most important thing I can do is to make other people feel better. While few of my friends knew that I had cancer (word was leaking out that I was sick), by

putting on the game face and having a positive attitude, I was helping them feel better about me.

We trekked around Europe for two weeks, on the streets of Rome
and Florence and the canals of Venice, to a barge through Bordeaux,
and on to Paris. From wine tasting to light hiking and riding bikes,
generous eating to sightseeing and floating along through small
towns on a barge, our days were full. In many ways, the therapy
of the trip was the best thing we could have done because it was a
last fling before the upcoming months that we could not have predicted by any forecast.

Upon returning home, we met with Dr. Khan to get our answer.
He told us that they had narrowed the possibilities down to a form
of leukemia but that he had not seen the final report from the lab.
He asked us to wait in his office while he went upstairs to the lab to
take a personal look at the slides so that he could personally confirm the diagnosis.

We could not let him leave without getting some additional
information, so we persisted. We asked him the range of options
we were looking at, and he divided them into two. The most serious case would be an acute form of leukemia, which would be quite
serious. That would mean that the leukemia was extremely active,
had come on suddenly, and would need immediate treatment. On
the other hand, if it were leukemia, a less serious outcome would be
a chronic form. In such a case, the leukemia could be managed on
a longer term basis and might not need to be managed as aggres-
sively. He said that there could be other diagnoses as well, but at
the moment he was leaning toward leukemia, although he did not
know whether it was acute or chronic and would need to review
the slides personally. Still, we would not let it end there. We always

wanted more information. He agreed to drive down deeper for a few more minutes and laid out the following:

Acute leukemia:
If it was an acute leukemia, we would probably begin with an intense round of inpatient chemotherapy. I would likely be hospitalized for a month at a time and would probably be facing three rounds of chemotherapy, with a week or so between each round. That would mean three months in the hospital. Most likely, the chemotherapy would bring about a remission, which would mean that at the end of the chemo-therapy less than 5 percent of my cells would be leukemia cells. However, for good measure I would undergo radiation treatments. In some circumstances, when a remission is not achieved by chemotherapy alone, patients must undergo a bone marrow or stem cell transplant, but we would discuss more about that much later.

Chronic Leukemia:
If the diagnosis was a chronic leukemia, the treatment would be much less aggressive. I would need many of the same protocols but they would not be as harsh. The chemo-therapy would be done as an outpatient. The drugs could be administered as oral drugs or a combination of oral and intravenous. The drugs would not be as strong and the side effects would not be as great, and a transplant may not be required at all.

With that, he left the room. We just looked at each other, stunned at what we'd heard. Once again, only time would tell. We had to wait for Dr. Khan to make a final diagnosis, and then which treatments he would order.

Leukemia? It had never occurred to us, and from what we knew about the disease, patients with leukemia usually have abnormal blood tests; my blood work was normal. How could it be? Four months of treatment? Were they crazy? How could anyone spend four months in the hospital? I had a very responsible position in Los Angeles and could not be away from it for that long. I could barely be away from the office for an afternoon, much less days, weeks, or months.

After nearly an hour, that seemed like an eternity, Dr. Khan returned to the exam room and confirmed that the tumors were not related to prostate cancer, but were a rare form of sarcoma, which presents itself as early-stage leukemia. However, it is rare because it does not show up in any blood tests. The tumors form outside the blood and bone marrow and attach to bone and ultimately work their way into the blood and marrow. It was called a granulocytic sarcoma that presents itself as acute myelogenous leukemia (AML). It was so rare that it affects only 1 percent of all patients diagnosed with AML (only about one hundred patients in the United States each year).

While AML is the most common form of leukemia, I was specifically diagnosed with extramedullary acute myelogenous leukemia.

That was Dr. Khan's diagnosis and the basis on which he was proceeding. However, the final diagnostic hurdle would come the next morning when the USC hematology team would meet, review the case with the pathology team, and arrive at a consensus.

Leukemia is a malignant liquid cancer of the bone marrow and blood. Other blood and marrow cancers include lymphoma and myeloma. Leukemia occurs due to the uncontrolled growth of blood cells and is classified as either acute leukemia or chronic leukemia. Within those two classes the leukemias break down further into classifications discussed later in this book and based on the types of cells that are involved. Mine was an acute form of leukemia, meaning that it came on rather suddenly and, as an acute illness, required immediate medical treatment in order to achieve a remission.

Chronic leukemias, on the other hand, take longer to develop, and patients can often go for years beyond diagnosis before receiving treatment.

The statistics below may help you understand the scope of leukemia:[6]

- An estimated thirty-five thousand new cases of leukemia are expected to be reported in the United States this year. Acute leukemias account for nearly 9 percent more of the cases than chronic leukemias. Most cases of acute leukemia occur in older adults; more than half of all cases occur after age sixty-four. Although it is often thought of as a disease that strikes children, leukemia strikes nine times as many adults as it does children. Approximately 30 percent of cancers in children ages zero to fourteen years are leu-

---

6   http://www.leukemia-lymphoma.org/all_page?item_id=9346

kemia, and leukemia is the most common form of death from cancer for young people.

- Men tend to be at slightly higher risks for leukemia than are women. In 2005, males were expected to account for more than 56 percent of the cases of leukemia. Sixteen men per one hundred thousand will be diagnosed with leukemia this year, and ten women per one hundred thousand will receive the same life-threatening news.

- Leukemia is one of the top fifteen most frequently occurring cancers in minority groups. Incidences of leukemia are highest among whites and lowest among American Indians and Alaskan natives. Leukemia rates are substantially higher for white children than for black children.

- Of the nearly thirty-five thousand new cases of leukemia, the distribution by type is expected to be:
  - Acute myelogenous leukemia (AML)—twelve thousand
  - Chronic lymphocytic leukemia (CLL)—eight thousand
  - Chronic myelogenous leukemia (CML)—four thousand six hundred
  - Acute lymphocytic leukemia (ALL)—four thousand

The balance is comprised of unclassified forms of leukemia.

Cancer is short for a series of horrible diseases. Leukemia, in my opinion (probably because I have it) is one of the toughest ones to deal with. Unlike organ cancers, for which there are surgical options, there is no such option because leukemia is a blood cancer, touching every part of your system that your blood reaches. What's more, the side effects and aftereffects can touch any part of the body as well and are extremely unpredictable and misunderstood. For instance, one major side effect is fatigue, which can last for months, years, or a lifetime. To this day, doctors do not know what causes it, how to predict it, or how to relieve it.

There in Dr. Khan's office that summer afternoon, we sat stunned; leukemia had never crossed our minds. And, tragically, Pamela's younger brother, Jerry, had succumbed to leukemia at the age of thirteen. It immediately brought back to her the nightmare of losing a loved one to the dreaded disease, although she also immediately understood that time, technology, and treatments had changed.

Dr. Khan told us that, based on looking at the slides personally, he was 100 percent positive of the diagnosis. Compounding the blow of the news was the fact that it was an acute form of leukemia, meaning that it was moving quickly and they needed to begin treatment immediately. But I had no idea how quickly they meant. I was sure I would have some time to straighten things out before getting started.

What we did not know for the moment was that "moving quickly" meant next week and that, by the following Monday afternoon, I would be in the hospital and, by that evening, I would be receiving the first drips of chemotherapy.

One of the hardest things to accept at the beginning was that I was sick at all. As I described earlier, I felt fine. I was not tired or fatigued beyond normal. Although under stress in my business life, it was not more than usual. I had no symptoms that caused me to complain to the doctors. All of my blood work was absolutely normal. I would not be talking to doctors or undergoing biopsies had it not been for the car accident and a few resulting tests. From being otherwise "normal" to being diagnosed with leukemia was an absolute shock that was nearly impossible to comprehend.

The diagnosis was difficult to come by because most leukemias turn up in blood tests. White blood cell counts are abnormal. Platelets may be too low. From a visually physical standpoint, a patient may bruise or bleed easily. Fatigue is a clue as well.

Extramedullary tumors can occur in the bone structures of the skull, sternum, ribs, vertebrae, pelvis, lymph nodes, and small intestine and around skeletal bones. In my case, tumors occurred in four locations: my vertebrae, my right arm, my right leg, and my prostate.

Thus, the ultimate diagnosis the doctors arrived at was that I had an extramedullary granulocytic sarcoma that presented itself with underlying acute myelogenous leukemia.

What a mouthful—and all for someone who felt fine. And, I did not have a history that suggested I was exposed to high risk for leukemia. High risk factors include:[7]

- Being male                                          Guilty
- Smoking, especially after sixty                      No
- Having had chemotherapy                              No
- Having had radiation therapy                         No
- Having had treatment for childhood leukemia          No

---

7   http://www.oncologychannel.com/leukemias/causes.shtml

- Exposure to atomic radiation                No
- Exposure to benzene                          Some
- Having a history of blood disorders         No

So, once again, I did not have the classic history that would make me a leukemia candidate. Nor did I have any of the symptoms. Beyond being male and having worked in a gas station as a teenager (with exposure to products that have benzene), I was not the classic presentation of a leukemia case.

But I soon learned that feeling fine had little to do with anything. I had leukemia, and I would have to answer the call to cancer. And I soon learned that leukemia is a serious disease that is life threatening despite the major advances in medicine over the past thirty years.

From a survival standpoint, significant progress has been made in recent years. The five-year survival rate has more than tripled in the past forty years for patients with leukemia. Between 1960 and 1963, a patient had a 14 percent chance of living for five years compared to those without leukemia (relative survival rate). By 1970–1973, the rate had jumped to 22 percent, and by 1995–2001, the overall relative survival rate was 48 percent. The survival rates differ by the age of the patient at diagnosis, gender, race, and type of leukemia.[8]

---

8   http://www.leukemia-lymphoma.org/all_page?item_id=9346

During 1996–2002 relative specific overall survival rates were:[9]

- Chronic lymphocytic leukemia (CLL): 74.2 percent
- Acute lymphocytic leukemia (ALL): 65.2 percent overall; 90.5 percent for children under five
- Chronic myelogenous leukemia (CML): 42.3 percent
- Acute myelogenous leukemia (AML): 20.4 percent overall; 53.1 percent for children under fifteen

At the present time there are approximately two hundred thousand people living with leukemia in the United States.

As the statistics show, my type of leukemia (AML), while the most common, has the lowest five-year survival rate and the highest number of deaths. And recent studies have shown that granulocytic sarcomas with AML have a lower complete remission rate and decreased remission duration.

So the die was cast, and none of the news we were finding was encouraging.

Statistics are fine, but every case is different. Each patient's course depends on the progression of the disease; the health and age of the patient; the type of transplant, if any; the risk factors the patient has encountered; the course of treatment; and many other factors.

You will learn that my treatment would be extremely difficult. I would undergo more inpatient chemotherapy than anyone I have met or spoken with who has had AML. I would spend more time in the hospital than any patient I would ever meet. My aftereffects

---

9    Ibid.

would be significant and there would be several occasions on which I would almost not survive.

Perhaps this is explained by the fact that I was over fifty when I was transplanted (most centers do not transplant patients over sixty, although the age continues to rise). Also, I would have a non-related transplant. We just don't know. What I know is that at one rough point Pamela would take Dr. Khan aside and tell him that she was strong and could take any news and wanted the truth about my prognosis. I would learn of this conversation much later (just previous to writing this book), and I would learn that he had told her that my prognosis was not good, given the acute nature of my disease and the fact that I would likely be dealing with an unrelated transplant.

## Getting Ready

I began to add the time up in my head. It was now August. I would need four months or more for my chemo, one month for radiation, and thirty days for the transplant, if I even needed to go that far. That was not so bad. With some luck, I would be able to be at the LA Chamber's annual inaugural dinner in January, 2004.

OK, I said, let's get going.

I did not know it then, but over the next few years I would observe nearly every major news event in the world (from the recall of California governor Gray Davis and the election of Arnold Schwarzenegger to the deaths of Ronald Reagan, Yassar Arafat, and Pope John Paul II and the election of Pope Benedict to political conventions and the unfolding of wars) and every major sporting event (among them the World Series, the Stanley Cup, the Super

Bowl, the Kentucky Derby, the Olympic Games, the NBA championship, the U.S. Open, the Masters, and the Final Four) from the confines of one of the six hospitals I would become acquainted with. The only major sports event I missed was World Cup Soccer, and that was only because it only occurs every four years.

The first stop after we'd finished with Dr. Khan was at the nurse's station. I would be admitted to the hospital the following Monday, so we needed blood and lab work immediately. Arrangements needed to be made. Authorizations from the insurance company had to be secured; a case like mine could run into the millions of dollars in cost. A myriad of details needed to be attended to. And all of this was before Pamela and I would have the time to process the news.

After a few hours of tests and processing, we were back in our car headed for home. It seemed as though the usual fifteen-minute ride took hours; we hit every stoplight. I don't recall specifically anything we may have said to each other. But once we arrived home the flood of details began to hit us. We were:

- Shocked
- Stunned
- Numb
- Scared

And when I use the word scared, it is the ultimate use of the word. There are many things that scare us in this life, but the thought of having cancer is probably one of the most frightening. Imagine being so frightened that you have time to consciously process the prospect that your life will soon end.

Now that we knew what we were dealing with, the time had come to make a few very difficult phone calls; the first calls were to Gerald and Jennifer. We told them that I had leukemia and gave them some general information but said that we would get together over the weekend and talk about all of the details.

We called Karen and Steve and let them know that we finally had an answer. Karen, in her usual way, went to work immediately and began research on the Internet. She set up an e-mail distribution list that would keep friends, family, and business associates in the loop about my progress. Little did we know at the time that this would prove to be one of the most valuable things that could be done for us.

We called my brothers, Pamela's family, and our friends and associates. I soon learned that it was as hard on the people receiving the news as it was for me to tell them. What could they say? How could they provide comfort?

We and our extended support system shared tears for several hours, and by early evening Pamela and I were alone together and emotionally exhausted, cuddling in bed as we pondered the future. Although we were physically alone, the last few hours had convinced us that we were being absorbed in a web of love and positive energy that we would need to harness in the months ahead.

Dr. Khan had made it clear that I would need the more extensive inpatient chemotherapy. We talked about how we would cope over the next month and how we could prepare for the treatment, which was scheduled to begin in just two days. It was a whirlwind discussion with few conclusions, mostly because we were so naïve about what to expect.

The chemotherapy that would begin the following Monday would come in two phases: induction and consolidation.

The goal of induction chemotherapy is to bring the disease into remission. Remission is when the patient's blood counts return to normal and bone marrow samples show no sign of active disease. Induction chemotherapy is very intense lasting longer and using much harsher drugs. Needless to say, the side effects are much harsher as well. If one round of treatment does not bring a remission, treatment may be repeated once or twice.

Successful induction chemotherapy destroys most of the leukemia cells, but a few will be left in the body. If these cells are not destroyed, they can cause a relapse of the disease.

The second phase of chemotherapy is called consolidation chemotherapy. The goal of consolidation chemotherapy is to destroy any remaining leukemia cells prior to embarking on radiation or a bone marrow or stem cell transplant.

We were most naïve about the side effects and risks of treatment at the various stages. When confronted with a life-threatening illness, you are suddenly facing an emergency.

Just cure me.

I realize today that we did not ask as many questions as we should have about what could possibly go wrong, what side effects I would endure (temporary and permanent). That is probably because it came upon us so quickly and we were urged to begin treatment immediately. We were simply in a daze and in a move-forward mindset. We just wanted to get going and did not want to hear anything else. I suppose that is what happens when your life is threatened out of nowhere.

In addition, except for facts about the chemotherapy, the doctors volunteered little information. After all, it was their job to save my life. Putting up with side effects or aftereffects was a distant second in their minds. So we knew little. They did tell us that this was a dangerous disease and that I would be undergoing what in many ways was a life-threatening round of treatment from which I might not recover. We understood this intellectually but truly had no idea what that meant—and certainly nothing with which to compare it. We had no idea that the treatment would actually take me to death's door, deliberately, before bringing me back to life.

The next day would be difficult as I would have to tell my coworkers at the office what was happening. The first thing in the morning I met with Marlee and told her everything we knew. I told her that I would need her now more than ever. She would have to take over many of my duties while I was in the hospital. We talked about people, organization, and priorities; she was a champ and agreed to do anything and everything she could. We had become friends over the past several years and, as you can imagine, our discussions were mixed with tears and hugs.

As an organizational president, I answered to a board of directors and needed to tell them as well. I began by calling George Kieffer to tell him that we finally had a firm diagnosis and treatment plan. He pledged his full support, as I knew he would, and asked me to call key members of the executive committee. After those discussions, all of which ended with pledges of support, I sent an e-mail to the entire board of directors and informed them of what was happening. At that point, my situation became news, given the public nature of my position.

Then I had to tell the staff. We brought the thirty-five people together and broke the news. We barely got through the tears—on both sides. Although we had only worked together for a few years, we had all become close. It was a very difficult meeting for all of them because I had kept the secret so close, and they were absolutely taken by surprise.

The rest of the day was devoted to wrapping things up at work and making sure that we had a plan for covering some of my duties that I would not be able to handle because I would be in the hospital. I would keep up on paperwork, phone calls, writing, and anything else I could handle in order to keep things as normal as possible. I had no idea how long I would be gone, just initially for a month or so, and I didn't have any idea what shape I would be in while hospitalized. Our planning was therefore tentative, and we would face things on a day-to-day basis.

That evening we flew up to San Jose to see some of our lifelong friends. Since we had no idea when we might see them again, this would be a last opportunity before the treatment and recovery onslaught would begin. It was a good day because we focused less on cancer than on our good times together. We flew home the next afternoon.

But before we left, we had an informal dinner party with many lifetime friends. It was a great evening that was capped off by one of the funniest episodes that would occur for several months.

At one point that evening, when the conversation lagged, Pamela turned to me and, in the most sincere manner, said, "I want you to look good when you go into the hospital, so let's go out and get you a haircut early in the morning before you go in." She was totally serious; she had forgotten that all of my hair would soon be gone thanks to the chemotherapy. We had a big laugh—one of the last we would have in a while.

On Sunday, Gerald and Jennifer came home, and we told them everything. We told them that leukemia was a serious disease and that my type was acute, which meant it was growing fast. We told them that I could die if we didn't get on it right away and that I would probably be in the hospital for several months. And we told them that it might turn out that the only thing that could save my life would be a bone marrow transplant.

They took it well—better than I'd expected. Some tears were shed, more mine than theirs. In fact they had more to say to me than I said to them. Their message was that I should stay strong; they knew I was strong enough to survive; they would be there for us every step of the way.

Although they were twins and were raised by the same parents in the same home under similar circumstances they turned out quite differently, and they handle situations differently. Gerald wears his emotions on his sleeve while Jennifer holds her emotions in and processes them in different ways.

I don't know how I handled it, although I have a clear recollection of a river of tears flowing down my face. I do have an exact recollection of where I was standing when I hugged them, the direction I was facing, and which one was in my right arm and which one was on my left. (Gerald was on the right and Jennifer on the left). After what seemed like an eternity, but was just a few ticks of the clock, Pamela put her arms around the three of us and we all collapsed in the living room. The emotion of the day and the prospects we faced in the days and months ahead were too much to face as the four of us hugged each other and pondered the future silently, together.

Gerald is ever the optimist and expresses that as well. He would be a tremendous source of inspiration for us—always looking on the bright side, always encouraging, and always giving me reasons to keep on moving forward. He would be my cheerleader, calling regularly to help me keep my spirits up. He would show his willingness to help by moving from his life in Orange County and living back home for six months.

Jennifer, on the other hand, is much more quiet and reserved. From the day she was born she has always analyzed things carefully. She would look at all details and ask questions until she was—and we were—blue in the face. She is much more introspective and reserved about expressing her emotions. When she would come to the hospital, more often than not, she would simply crawl into bed with me and we would hug and talk. At that point in her life, she had been accepted to graduate school at the distinguished University of Chicago Harris School of Public Policy. She would decide that she wanted to be closer to the family and defer her admission—a great personal sacrifice. After Gerald had spent time at home, she would move back as well to be of help.

The balance of Sunday was a blur. More phone calls. Sorting mail and prioritizing things that needed to be done. More walks through the neighborhood. More quiet time alone contemplating an uncertain future.

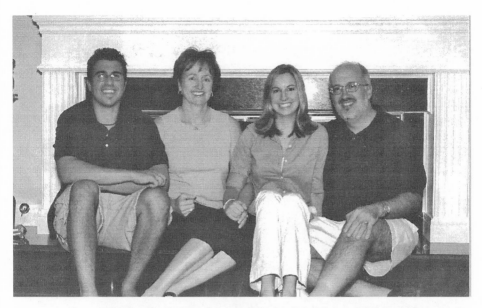

The family gathered around for a photo the evening
before chemotherapy began. Photo by Marlee Miller.

That evening we sat around the house and talked until late in the evening. Some friends joined us to help us get our minds off of the events that would come. We talked about good times we'd had together and about how encouraged we should be that my doctor had caught my disease when he had. Not expecting that it would happen, we enjoyed one of the heartiest laughs we would have in months.

Monday, August 18, 2003, came too soon. We were due at the hospital at 9:00 a.m. The USC Norris Cancer Center was only a few minutes away from home, and we left at 8:58 a.m. After all, I would be there for a month; there was no need to be there a minute more than necessary.

After the check-in process was over, it was time to get started. First in line were more blood tests, tests for vital signs, etc., in the outpatient treatment area. Then I was off to a small room for my first bone marrow biopsy. It is a necessary procedure that all leukemia patients must undergo; unfortunately, it is also one that is painful and is generally not done under anesthesia. The bone marrow biopsy, also known as a bone marrow aspiration, is a test that is designed to obtain a sample from bone marrow to determine the extent to which leukemia cells are present in the marrow.

I was placed on my stomach and prepped for the sterile procedure, with Pamela in the room sitting beside me. A small amount of local anesthetic injected into the skin at the site of the biopsy was the only anesthesia used. It was a very painful procedure.

I did not see much of what was happening, but the bottom line is that Dr. Khan inserted a tool through my skin and into my hip to obtain a core sample of bone. Think of it as though the doctor is opening a bottle of wine. He or she inserts the corkscrew in my hip and turns it until the cork is fully pierced and then removes it. Take it from me; removing a wine cork is much easier!

Pamela watched the process and told me later that it was a horrific and barbaric scene. Dr. Khan was perched over me, all of his six foot three frame, with tools in hand. She told me that he got up on his toes and bore down into my hip with all of his strength, driving the instrument into my bones until he was able to get a sample. But it did not end there. Not until several samples were taken, and I had uttered more curses in pain than I remembered having done in my lifetime, was he done.

The next step was to get some heart studies done, the most significant being a heart function test called a multiple gated acquisition (MUGA) scan. The doctors needed to determine how well my heart was performing and whether it could withstand the stress of the chemotherapy and radiation treatments I was about to undergo. To do this, they measured my ejection fraction. When the left ventricle of the heart contracts, forcing blood out into the body, it's called ejection since it is ejecting the blood out into the arteries. The left ventricle doesn't pump out all of the blood, so that there is always a small amount of blood remaining for the next contraction, and that is that fraction that the scan measures.

Doctors like to see an ejection fraction of not less than 55 percent. Mine was just under the target, but not enough to cause a major concern.

Then I was off to receive my first catheter.

A catheter is a thin, flexible tube that can be placed in a vein, artery, organ, or body cavity and is used as a path for administering drugs, food products, blood, and blood products, and for withdrawing fluids from the body. Blood samples can also be removed through catheters. The placement of the catheters was not a terribly painful procedure compared to other things I would go through, and the catheters would save me what amounted to be hundreds, maybe thousands, of needle sticks. Little did I know, I would receive three different types of catheters and have a total of more than fifteen insertions during my journey.

The first catheter I received was called a peripherally inserted central catheter, or "PICC line," a thin, long, soft plastic tube that functions as an intravenous (IV) line. PICC lines are inserted under a local anesthetic by a nurse who inserts the line into a large vein in the arm and guides the catheter up into the main vein near the heart. An X-ray is taken to assure that the catheter is in the right location.

After the PICC was placed, I was then off to my room.

But having a PICC line is not as easy as the insertion alone. Since the catheter is an opening into the body, it is ripe for infection (I would have a few—they are hard to avoid). Every day the nurses, Pamela, or I had to clean the dressing and flush the line with a syringe of heparin or normal saline (used to break up any blood clot that may have formed in the line). In addition, I couldn't get the catheter wet, which made showering difficult.

But it was worth the price to avoid the needles.

I would gain experience with two other types of catheters, the next being a Hickman catheter. A Hickman catheter is a long plastic or rubber tube that is inserted into one of the main blood vessels that lead to the heart. It can be a single port, a double port, or triple port (ports are openings used for administering or withdrawing fluids). I always had double lumen Hickman catheters. The Hickman catheter was done under a general anesthetic. As my doctor explained in advance, he would make two small incisions, one near the collarbone, and one between my nipple and breastbone. The catheter would be tunneled under the skin between these two incisions and threaded into a vein in my chest.

When I had my central line placed, it was done in a similar manner, except it was done by a surgeon under a local anesthetic and placed just above the heart. A central line requires about the same level of maintenance and cleaning as the Hickman and the PICC lines.

Now that the preliminaries had been taken care of it was time to proceed to my room in the bone marrow transplant unit.

In the days just prior to my admission, my mind went wild about the road ahead. What would chemotherapy be like? How sick would I get? When would I lose my hair (the answer to that question was answered two weeks into chemo when I awoke to a pillow full of hair)? Was the hospital food any good? Would I get along well with the nurses? How could I possibly stand to be in the hospital for a month at a time? What kind of room would I have? How could I be apart from friends, family, and work for so long? Would I ever be able to come home?

The answers to these questions, and many others, would all come in due time.

The first answer nearly broke me.

I was certain that the hospital room would be nothing like I had ever seen. After all, I would be there for a month or more at a time and I was sure they had to make it comfortable. I imagined a room much like the modern pregnancy suites with an oversized bed, soothingly-painted walls, home-like furniture, and room to accommodate the family. I could not have been more wrong!

Instead, I was placed in a stark, white-painted, drab, tiny room with more monitoring equipment than you could shake the proverbial stick at. There was room for one chair and little else. Of course, a typically uncomfortable hospital bed took up most of the room.

I was devastated. I was sure that they did not expect me to live there for a month. How could they expect that? Was this any way to treat a patient with a terminal illness?

Pamela stayed with me for a while until the hour grew late.

The first thing she did was to climb into bed with me. We cuddled for a few minutes until a nurse came in and told us it was against hospital policy. That was a policy we would ignore; Pamela would climb into bed with me many more times—it was the only real human contact I would have.

To hell with policy.

Pamela sensed that something was wrong, but I would be the last one to admit any disappointment or sadness. It was time to put on my game face—a face that I would need to wear many times during this journey. After all, I was the one who needed to be strong for her, for my family, and for my friends. I could not show any sign of weakness. That was a decision I made early on because sometimes you need to fight, not for yourself, but for your friends and family who are fighting for and supporting you.

*As I Lay Me Down to Sleep*[10]

As I lay me down to sleep this I pray; that you will hold me dear
I'll whisper your name into the sky and I will wake up happy.
—Sophie B. Hawkins

After Pamela left, I sat on the bed and cried like a baby for what seemed like hours. It would not be the first time I cried through the evening. It did not matter whether the days were sunny or the nights were rainy. The feeling of loneliness, the surge of emotions, and the uncertainty of it all was ever present.

Hawkins's words do not overstate the feelings that were in my heart every night. It is not possible to overstate how lonely it was every night as the lights would go out—how I would pray to myself that Pamela, my children, and my loved ones would hear my voice and that tomorrow would be a better day.

---

10   http://www.lyricscafe.com/h/hawkins_sophieb/016.htm

I would not understand it until much later, but I would come to realize that the hospital room needed to be the way it was. I suppose I was under the false assumption that I was going in for simple procedures; after all, the doctors simplified them for me. I was not aware of the fact that I would be exposed to life-threatening situations that would require heroic medical intervention. Nor did I know that I needed all of the provisions of critical care immediately at my disposal. I would soon learn these things and would understand why the room needed to be as it was. Nevertheless, the room was a major disappointment when I first saw it, and it did not give me a warm feeling about the months to come.

Here is how I captured the first day in the hospital in my journal:

August 18, 2003

Today began as one of the most difficult in my life. After doing some paperwork at the house and saying good-bye to the dogs (more emotional than I imagined), we went to Norris. After checking in at the hospital, I had a MUGA scan—a test to measure my heart output. That required a few injections—the outcome was that my heart was in good shape. Following the scan I was to have a PICC line inserted, but the timing was fouled up and I spent the next few hours in the Day Hospital, mostly sleeping. There were lots of other blood tests as well throughout the day, so I slept in between all of those. It seems as though that will become my routine. Pamela and I were exhausted from all of the stress of the trip to San Jose. The line was finally inserted by late afternoon. It was somewhat painful and uncomfortable, but it went as well as could be expected.

We saw Dr. Khan and he went through the treatment plan once again. He took Pamela aside and spoke with her privately. Gerald came to the hospital and gave me a card. The words he wrote made me cry; he is always so expressive. I will save it, along with Pamela's and Jenny's forever. We were then taken to Room 304 in the Bone Marrow Unit—my home for the next several weeks.

Honestly, I was crushed. It is a very small room and looks like an ICU unit. I tried not to cry, but it hit me like a ton of bricks. It just looks like such a sick place, and I am having a hard time imagining me being here as long as I need to be.

We met the staff; Dr. Tony Talebi, and Lisa Mark, N.P. They were great and answered all of our questions. We settled in, and after Pamela and Gerald left for a while, dinner was served. To my surprise, it was not that bad.

Pamela and Gerald returned, and we talked about her visit with Dr. Khan. I learned that things were more serious than I thought. They discovered that the leukemia had invaded the bone marrow. Tough news. We cried even more but I must say that Gerald handled things very well and is an excellent source of strength and support for us for such a young man.

As I got ready for bed I know that I/we are embarking on yet another journey. I know it won't be easy on any of us and I am especially worried about Pamela, Gerald, and Jennifer. I know that this will be a tough battle and today's news doesn't make things any easier, but the fight begins right here, right now. We all have so much to live for and we must beat this.

## Chemo Round 1

I dozed on and off to the sounds of the television and the machines in my room. I would soon get used to those machines, but that first night I thought I could not sleep with them. Soon enough I would not be able to sleep without their noise. I was hooked up to several IVs that supplied fluids and medications to me, and every time a line would become kinked or clogged up the machine would set off a loud beeping alarm. Of course, the alarm would need to be loud enough for the nurse to hear it at the station, and I would wake up.

Here is the entry from the second day of my journal:

August 19

Shortly after midnight two nurses came into my room and, to my surprise, told me that they were going to begin my chemo in a few moments. I did not know it would start that soon and was somewhat taken by surprise. I had imagined that the doctors would be there, that perhaps I would be taken to a special room, that there would be special protocols, etc. No, they said it would happen right there in my room. No need for my wife to be there; it was no big deal. But for them, a few moments turned into two hours. At about 2:00 a.m. they came in with the chemicals and went through the routine. After going through their multi-checking procedures, they hooked the chemo bags up to my PICC, opened the line, and my treatments were underway. I didn't feel a thing. I just dozed off to sleep, finally, but scared as I could be.

After getting chemo I was awakened at 5:00 a.m. to begin my day! I called Pam an hour later to tell her that I was receiving the chemo. We both cried, and she said she would be there as soon as she could. I watched TV, read and responded to e-mail, did some writing for the chamber, and went through my morning routine. The phone calls started from friends and colleagues, although I didn't feel much like talking.

During the day I was visited by a social worker. She asked me to fill out a form on which I was to circle how I felt on a scale of 1–10 about various things like my prognosis, money, spiritual care, and other stuff. I call it the "smiley face" form.

Pam is having a hard time; I worry so much about her. We took two short walks in the hallway. It was a good time amidst all of the agony. We spoke with Dr. Khan about starting to test my brothers for compatibility, and he said that could wait. We were puzzled but dropped the matter.

It was the end of my first full day and, although the physical side effects were only beginning, one side effect had taken a full grip—loneliness. I know the fight is in me, but I don't know how I can be cooped up in here.

The biggest challenge of the day was to tell Jenny that they found cells in the marrow. My chances for survival had dropped, and she took it very hard. She climbed in bed with me and we cried and hugged each other as Pamela tried to mask her emotions while sitting in the chair. I encouraged Jenny to talk with Gerald and with friends and to stay positive because I was.

As she left she went to the white board in my room and wrote the words that stayed there as long as I was in Norris:

LOVE YOU DADDY,   ♡   JENNY

Despite my introduction to Norris, I have no criticism of the facility or its staff as I reflect on the experience. It is a good hospital and I have good things to say about the people.

The bone marrow transplant (BMT) unit is a small, five-bed unit. I knew every nurse and every doctor. I received excellent attention. If I hit the call button, one of the nurses was there in seconds. And Norris had the best hospital food. It was a nurturing environment, with nurses who really cared about me and my family; we became a family together. It was truly a cocooning environment that cared for us and all of our needs.

I knew that I would need to resolve within myself to try and keep my life in the hospital as normal as possible. I would keep up with what was happening at the office as best I could.

Foremost among those duties was writing a weekly public policy column I developed for the chamber called "The Business Perspective." This became an award-winning and widely distributed opinion piece on public issues facing LA, California, and the country. (Incidentally, throughout all of my treatment I never missed writing a weekly column, with help of the staff.) The motivation to keep the streak alive gave me energy—both physical and mental. If I had not had the mental challenge of working and writing, it would have been easy to shrivel up as much mentally as I was physically. I would keep things as normal as possible and avoid sympathy.

We tried to make my room look like home. Family photos were everywhere. Pamela brought my special pillow and hung inspirational messages. Karen supplied her special touches and made me a special blanket—all things to make the place look less like a hospital and more like home.

Little did I know how difficult it would be to do that.

I quickly learned that clocks mean nothing in a hospital. When the nurses were ready to do their work, they were ready, and it did not matter whether it was midnight or 4:00 a.m. They would start treatments and testing at their convenience, not mine. This was another rule I would learn to live by.

Chemo started around midnight. Susan, my first nurse, carried with her the toxic chemotherapy drugs that would begin the process of killing as many cells as it could attack—both those that were stealing my life as well as those that were keeping me alive. The unfortunate thing about chemo is that it does not discriminate. It kills the good cells along with the bad. Throughout my treatment, I received six chemotherapy drugs (Ara-C, Idarubicin, high-dose Ara-C, Fludarabine, Melphalan, and Methotrexate).

Administering chemotherapy is a highly regulated procedure. To begin with, not just any nurse can administer chemotherapy. The nurse must have a specific license and certification as a chemo nurse. As they were before the administration of all drugs, nurses were required to check my wristband to make sure that I was the person for whom the drug was prescribed. They always had to ask my date of birth as well. But with chemotherapy, a second licensed chemotherapy nurse was required to do the same—it was an important double check that I soon learned they would forgo once they knew me well enough. The nurses were gowned, masked, and gloved to protect them from accidental spills. Any spillage of the chemo could be toxic—or at least painful—to them.

However, I thought it was odd that I was not gowned or gloved; I was only protected by my sheets. The chemo would be dripping in the tubes all around me, and if a tube had broken, I could have become contaminated; I had no protection. It was, indeed, a strange irony. Perhaps the licensing authorities should look at that.

The chemo drugs were kept in a bag, hung from an IV pole, and connected to a pump that whirred all night (and kept me awake) and beeped loudly if the line became clogged (or if I somehow fell asleep and the line became twisted or kinked). The pump sent the drugs through the line, into the catheter, and into my veins. The bag needed to be shielded from light in a darker bag and had to be checked every half hour to make sure it was flowing properly.

Unfortunately, the lines got clogged or kinked often. When this happened, the pumps sensed the situation and shut down. But that is not all they did; the pumps gave out an ear-piercing sound loud enough that it could be heard in the nurse's station so that they could come to the room to resolve the problem. If it was loud enough to be heard down the hall, imagine how loud it was at the bedside. Blaring! And it was enough to wake me up constantly.

I received little education at that point about what to expect. How long would it take to feel the effects of the drugs? Would I get sick right away? What would I feel? Nothing asked, nothing volunteered. So I just laid there waiting for the ball to drop on me for the next four hours. Nothing happened immediately, but by the time I fell asleep it was nearly 5:00 a.m.; I had been up for nearly twenty-four hours. An hour later the nurses were back, taking blood samples and getting ready for the day.

This was just the beginning of the long journey.

One of the lessons I learned that first evening was that I was no longer in control of my life in the hospital. There would be almost no time when I did not hear machines of all types blaring out and interfering with sleep. Nurses or medical assistants would usually wake me every few hours to take my blood pressure or temperature—or to weigh me!

I never understood why they needed to know how much I weighed at 3:00 a.m.

Nor did I understand why they need to clean the bathroom in the middle of the night, much less why they need to turn the lights on in the room when they clean the bathroom. Why not just turn on the lights in the bathroom, close the door, and be as quiet as possible? I guess that is too logical.

If I had a dollar for every time I had my temperature or blood pressure taken over the last few years, I would be a rich man today.

I discovered that there is absolutely no predictability in the course of treatment. Blood tests were taken every few hours at first, then a few times a day. As my blood counts would improve, it would seem as though we were making progress, but at times we were lulled into a false sense of security, and we found that things could turn on a dime. I would get good blood numbers one day and bad numbers the next. I would feel well enough to get out of bed one day and walk the halls, and by the evening would have high fevers and be barely able to move. We just never knew. I would see the same thing in other patients. Some would do well for a day then collapse. Others would have rough days every day. It was so uncertain and so random. So while I trace through the steps that we went through, just know that one thing is certain—the effects of chemotherapy will be different for each patient.

As I mentioned earlier, I also learned that time in the hospital would not be my own. I could not plan on anything. Doctors, nurses, and technicians could come in at any time and expect that I would immediately drop what I was doing. It did not matter whether I was having a private conversation or whether I was doing some serious writing. They would expect that I would immediately drop what I was doing so that they could do what they wanted. No advance notice; little patience. That was simply the way it was.

There would be a dizzying array of tests and procedures that could be ordered at any time and, as I said before, I would be called on when they were ready, not when it fit my schedule or how I felt at the time. I would even be awakened from a deep sleep to take a simple diagnostic test.

Privacy?

As they say. Forget about it.

As much as I obsessed about waiting for the effects of chemotherapy, nothing happened for several days. I continued to receive
treatments but had no side effects. I was told that some people react
well to chemo and, so far I was in that boat. It looked like it would
be a piece of cake.

Then, on the fourth day, the storm hit.

Lance Armstrong, the famous world champion cyclist who
came back from testicular caner to win Tour de France seven times
described chemotherapy by saying "chemo felt like a kind of living
death. I would lie in bed half asleep, and lose track of time, including whether it was day or night—and I didn't like that."[11]

I don't want to scare you by using his characterization; that is
true in the worst of cases. But it is a treatment that is capable of
making you seriously ill before it makes you better. It is important
that you understand how bad it can be so that you are prepared if it
happens or relieved and encouraged if it does not.

The effects are somewhat predictable and, unfortunately, I had
most of them. First, I experienced something that closely resembled
"Montezuma's Revenge." Since the chemo kills cells with little dis-
crimination, including bacteria, the good cells die and give way to
diarrhea. I had it bad. It was so bad that I became extremely weak
and unable to get out of bed for long stretches. Nurses needed to
help me to the bathroom or to portable commodes. At times I was
so weak that they had to clean me. It was an emasculating experience in which I lost all dignity.

11    Lance Armstrong, *It's Not About the Bike* (New York: G.P. Putnam's Sons, 2000),
      135

This was complicated by a related effect at the other end—nausea. And, once you get into that cycle, eating anything is a chore that only reminds you that everything you eat has to come out, so it's is no longer a priority. These side effects robbed me of valuable nutrition and electrolytes and just made me feel that much worse. And it required that I receive intravenous nutrition to keep my nutrition levels adequate.

In addition to these side effects, the chemo sapped my strength at all levels. I did not feel like doing anything. There were times I had high fevers, only to be followed by chills. I would sleep for hours, followed by periods of insomnia. There were times when I would not want to see anyone. I would become irritable. I would lose my normally good sense of humor and just not be myself.

Chemo also takes away your strength. By causing diarrhea and nausea and taking away your appetite, it causes your nutrition levels to fall and the intravenous levels do not take the place of regular meals. When you get out of bed and try to walk the halls and get some exercise the strength just is not there; forget about the stamina.

During the chemo period, the nurses monitored my blood counts at least several times a day. They needed to keep a close watch on the number of white blood cells, which fight infection; red cells, which give energy; and platelets, which control bleeding because one of the side effects of chemotherapy is that the counts will decline. As these counts declined, I would receive transfusions of various blood and blood products to make sure that the counts did not get too far out of balance; if they were too far out of balance my health would be at risk.

Unfortunately, the first major complications occurred almost immediately. This one was related to my platelet level.

Normal platelet counts range from one hundred fifty thousand to four hundred thousand. Platelets play a vital role in the blood clotting process by forming a platelet plug. Single platelets bind to the site of a wound and then the platelets adhere to each other. The result is that they bind together to stop the bleeding. This allows the wound to heal.

Leukemia patients often have low platelet levels, and the chemotherapy further destroys them, making bleeding a high risk. The chemotherapy and related drugs are expected to bring platelet levels down—but seldom to less than twenty thousand. If the count drops below that, the patient needs platelet transfusions. But mine sank to extremely low levels—at times to less than five thousand and often to under one thousand or immeasurable.

This became a dangerous risk for me for two reasons. First, with platelet levels at or below five thousand, I could start bleeding internally by simply bumping myself on a bedrail. I could have an internal bruise or be bleeding internally and not even know it until it was too late. The other issue was that I had somehow developed antibodies that were rejecting the platelets I had been given. The form of rejection caused me to go into severe respiratory paralysis and distress to the point where I was unable to breathe. If we did not find a compatible donor soon, we would have major problems because my system would reject the platelets that were being administered and I would likely bleed to death.

The doctors tried to determine why I had these antibodies. Generally, women who had been through childbirth and people who had received prior blood transfusions could have a similar antibody profile that I exhibited. But I said that I was not in either category; then Pamela reminded me that I had received transfusions at birth from the unwinding of my umbilical cord. And some of the transfusions were likely from nurses who'd had children. The mystery was solved, but the problem still existed.

The first time I had a reaction, I was being attended to by a nurse who was not a part of the regular Norris staff. As I began to have labored breathing and went into convulsions, Pamela found the nurse and brought her into the room. She panicked. The nurse ran out of the room, screaming, "I didn't do anything; it's not my fault." She grabbed her purse from the nurses' station and ran out of the hospital. We never saw her again. Fortunately, Pamela kept her cool and found the doctors and nurses and they administered medications that calmed the distress and resolved the situation.

But the next step was to find platelets that my body would not reject. After Pamela told the doctors about my transfusions at birth, they suggested that there was the possibility that one of my siblings could match me. Fortunately, we discovered that my brother, Lee, had platelets that were compatible with me, and he flew to LA many times (courtesy of Southwest Airlines) to give me the platelets I needed.

Through the process with the platelets, we learned that the blood supply system in this country is far from patient friendly, to put it mildly. Nor is it consistent from city to city or from hospital to hospital. I have great respect for the Red Cross and the work it does in disaster situations, but the response we received from at least one of their branches was anything but acceptable. Nor was it consistent from one branch to the other when it came to blood issues. While this may not be generally true, the centers we worked with in

California worked normal business hours, and patients' needs do not follow these hours. If you needed blood products outside these hours and your center was closed, you lost. And platelets have a very short shelf life (just a few days), so platelets donated late in the week are of no use by Monday! The process to get blood or platelets was bureaucratic—often taking too long. And their restrictions were so complicating that they presented a threat to my survival.

For example, my brother, Lee, lived in northern California, and we were in Los Angeles. But getting the arrangements made to draw blood, test it, and ship it, often took way too long. In fact, one Friday evening I was in desperate need of platelets from Lee, and they threatened to delay shipping until the following Monday even though the hospital had followed the protocols and paperwork in complete detail. We even proposed signing a release that would absolve the blood bank of any liability in sending my brother's blood outside of their normal procedures, which they rejected. It was not until the doctors and Pamela got on the phone and demanded action that action was taken. Without it, my survival was in serious jeopardy. Fortunately, we got action, but on other occasions, we could not take the risk and simply flew Lee to LA.

My chemo also allowed me to see what I would look like without any hair. I had been losing my hair for years. After a few weeks, I learned that I did not have any moles or indentations on my head and that I would not look so bad if I lost all of my hair. What a relief!

Mouth care is critical with chemo patients because the chemotherapy acts first on fast-growing cells, and mouth cells are among the fastest growing due to the moisture in the mouth. The mouth sores were so severe that I could barely swallow saliva, much less food, for days at a time. Mouth rinses occurred with regularity, every few hours.

The chemotherapy also caused violent headaches. Unfortunately, these side effects were par for the course and little could be done about them. Imagine having headaches so bad that you needed to take medication and then having mouth sores that were so severe that you could not even swallow water to take pills. It was a vicious cycle. It got to the point where I was placed on a self-controlled (within limits) morphine drip.

After about two weeks, I reached a predictable but low point in the chemo routine. I became neutropenic, which means that my white blood cell levels were at their lowest and I was most susceptible to infection. Neutropenia is the term used to describe the condition when your neutrophil count in your blood is too low. A neutrophil is a type of white blood cell that kills bacteria. White blood cells are the cells in your body that fight infections or germs. The bone marrow produces these cells along with other types of blood cells. Neutrophils are the first line of defense when your body needs to fight an infection, so they are monitored closely. Think of them as knights in shining armor coming to rescue you from an infection or germ.

Once I was neutropenic, I needed to be fully isolated, and anyone who visited needed to be gloved, masked, and gowned. I needed special food dictated by what is called a low microbial diet (see Appendix D). This food needed to be specifically treated; even my ice was involved (it had to be made from distilled water). There could be no risk of infection because, given my low blood counts, an infection could be fatal to me.

I recall waking up that first morning after neutropenia set in. The nurse came into the room fully gowned and gave me the news. But I knew before she said a word. I had done enough reading to know that something had changed; her gown and mask said more than words can convey. About an hour later, Pamela came to see me, gowned, masked, and gloved. There would be no kissing or hugging—no direct contact—for ten days to two weeks until my blood counts recovered. I took one look at her in her astronaut-like outfit and cried like a baby.

Despite the precautions, the risks of Chemo Phase 1 were hardly over.

During this first major crisis, Pamela reached out to a good friend, John Bryant. A charismatic community leader in LA, John came to my room several times to pray with us. And he had Dr. Cecil Murray, the senior pastor of the First African Methodist Episcopal (A.M.E.) Church in LA, call on the phone to pray with us as well. It did not matter that we were of different religions (to any of us); we needed prayers from all. The complications were just beginning.

I began to experience severe stomach pain which, was diagnosed as typhlitis. Typhlitis is an inflammation of the stomach. Patients with anemia, AIDS, lymphoma, kidney transplants, cytomegalovirus, and other malignancies have been known to acquire typhlitis, which I did as well. Typhlitis is a major complication that, more often than not, is fatal—especially to someone with a compromised immune system like me. Fortunately, the doctors got on it right away and, although it was touch and go for several days, I became one of the success stories.

It wasn't that easy; I am told that I hovered near death for a few days with both high and low blood pressure, high fevers, and related complications.

Unfortunately, the infection process, combined with the chemotherapy, put great stress on my heart, and I developed congestive heart failure and atrial fibrillation (A-fib). My heart was under stress and was doing the job as well as it could, but it just could not keep up with the demands.

Irregular, rapid beating of the atrial chambers of the heart is what indicates atrial fibrillation. This happens when the normal system that conducts electricity in the heart does not function properly. A storm of electrical activity causes them to fibrillate hundreds of times per minute. The A-fib was causing my heart to beat in a rapid and irregular manner. I would have heart rates of one hundred fifty to two hundred, rather than a more normal seventy to eighty beats per minute.

This can result in varying symptoms from relatively mild ones, such as fatigue and cough, to serious ones, such as angina and stroke. Of the 700,000 people in the United States who suffer strokes each year, [12]approximately 15 percent are caused by atrial fibrillation.[13]

Whether atrial fibrillation happens at high or low heart rates, its irregular rhythm means the ventricles can't pump blood efficiently to the rest of the body. Instead, blood pools in the heart and the body doesn't get enough blood as quickly as it demands.

When I had my first A-fib episode, the cardiologists talked about what to do. There were several options that included medications, ablating (cauterizing) areas of the heart where the A-fib was origi-

12   http://www.cbsnews.com/stories/2005/06/09/health/main700773.shtml
13   http://www.americanheart.org/presenter.jhtml?identifier=4451

nating and implanting a pacemaker, and a procedure called cardioversion (using electricity to shock the heart back to a normal
sinus rhythm). What they meant was that they wanted to perform
the cardioversion option. Cardioversion essentially involves the
use of defibrillator paddles to shock the heart back into a normal
rhythm—much like when doctors start a heart that has stopped
beating.

I was just recovering from typhlitis and not feeling well. Then
the A-fib came on, and I could feel my heart pounding inside of
me, causing some pain and lots of distress. The doctors came in
(Pamela was not there at the time) and were speaking among themselves as though I was not even in the room. That happened a lot.
In tones that were not exactly hushed, they said they thought they
should "fry" me, using that specific word.

I recall specifically moaning and saying, "Nobody is going to fry
me." Within thirty minutes, Pamela arrived for her daily visit. I told
her what had happened, and the next thing I knew Pamela asked
the doctor to step outside my room.

Once outside my room she told the doctor that her choice of
words was inappropriate and that she should never use such words
around any patient whether she thought the patient could hear her
or not. Somewhat facetiously she asked the doctor whether "frying"
was a medical term and admonished her that she had no business
using such words or in any way frightening a patient—especially
her husband! Pamela told the doctor that if she ever spoke around
me again in those terms or in any way tried to frighten us, she
would demand that the doctor be removed from my case.

It was a learning experience for the doctor, and she eventually
apologized.

It worked. No frying. Medications brought the situation under control.

Within a few short weeks, by necessity, Pamela had gone from a quiet and gentle person to a real tiger; she was my advocate, who spoke up for me and for us and would not let anyone walk over us or take advantage of our vulnerable situation. I am so thankful she was there for us.

After spending so much time in the hospital, mostly in bed and unable to get around and exercise, I began to develop even greater severe back pain and muscle atrophy. It may have been new pain from being in bed for so long or it may have been an exaggeration of my prior back problems. The morphine drip was extremely effective in combating both the back pain and the headaches, but it left me drugged and drowsy.

I tried Dilaudid, which caused me to hallucinate. Other narcotics worked well but the side effects were not acceptable either. My doctors and I experimented with pain patches and other oral medications. But little seemed to work. It was another hurdle that would plague me in the months ahead.

The problem was that I began to slide down a slippery slope. I was beginning to become deconditioned very early in my treatment. Due to my back pain and muscle tone, as well as my susceptibility to fainting and infections, I was losing strength. I could not walk or get adequate exercise. This would be a problem that would plague me in the years ahead.

I don't remember how many times over the next several weeks I received various tests. I know there were chest X-rays every week and blood tests at least twice a day. Physical therapists came by twice a day. I took walks around the unit with Pamela, Gerald, and

Jennifer when I was strong enough. But I could not go outside or go near an open window for fear of infection. I had some contact with nearly every medical specialty. Since USC is a teaching hospital, I was seen by medical students, residents, and fellows so that they could learn about my case, ask questions, and impress the attending physicians.

Curiously enough I was seldom seen by the social workers to see how I was doing from an emotional perspective.

The chemotherapy experience was all that I'd worried it could be. I experienced extreme side effects like the usual ones that people talk about. But the abnormal ones like A-fib, typhlitis, and others I have described raised many red flags about the perils of upcoming chemo rounds that gave me great cause for concern. But I knew that we had no choice; we had to keep moving forward despite knowing that, in all likelihood, we might see reruns in the weeks and months to come of what we had just been through.

But the time to go home for the first time was soon upon us. After nearly six weeks in the hospital, my blood counts had returned to an acceptable level, the typhlitis was beaten back, and my heart was under control. I was able to go home—for five days.

The thing I remember most was leaving the hospital in a wheelchair and waiting for our car outside of the hospital for but a few minutes. I sat there in the wheelchair, too weak to walk, and felt the warmth of the sun on my face and fresh air across my lips for the first time since my admission. I must say that there were times when I thought I would never experience these feelings or smell the sweet odor of the flowers again.

We got in for the brief ride home, and I cried again. I did not know whether I would ever take this ride again, and I was so thankful that we were underway.

It was great to be home, if only for a few days. Seeing the house, the dogs (Connie and Brandon—two of the best golden retrievers you would ever meet), our room, and most of all sleeping in bed with Pamela was a welcome break, even though I was miserably weak. I slept for many hours at a time. I was unable to do anything for myself. But finally I was home.

For the short week at home, we had to be extra careful. Although I was no longer neutropenic, I needed to maintain the low-microbial diet as well as the cleanliness and food washing procedures.

It was our first exposure to what was involved in Pamela being a caregiver; and as we would soon learn, it was only the tip of the iceberg. Since I had little strength and was always napping or resting in my chair, I relied on her for *everything*. In addition to assisting me with simply getting around in the house and keeping track of all of the details of our everyday life, the cooking and food burden became hers as well.

The first task was to become acclimated. Being gone from home for over a month made everything strange. Sure, I knew everything. The dogs knew me. I recognized the smells. But I was like a stranger in my own home. I had to get used to things all over again. It only took a few hours again for me to become comfortable, but it was not instantaneous.

And the mail had piled up while I was gone. Soon the financial reality of our situation hit when I began to review bills from the hospital and notices from the insurance company. I won't give the name of the company, but it was clear from looking at their reports that they were more interested in rejecting claims than in paying them. In earlier times in my career, I had worked in human resources, and I knew a lot about health care and insurance coverage, so I called the company to discuss the situation. Most of what I heard on the phone from customer service representatives was simply nonresponsive, so I called in a supervisor.

Supervisors were no help either. They blamed the situation on improper billing codes by the hospital and doctors. They said that some things were not covered and scared us. It was always someone else's fault.

I tried to tell them that I had just returned home from chemotherapy and was facing months of intense treatments. I had leukemia and simply could not sort this out. I respectfully asked if they could assign a case manager to help us out with this. I was so emotional about the situation that I began crying on the phone—helpless and in need of a caring human being.

The supervisor I was talking to said no; it was my responsibility.

It was no way to treat a patient with a life-threatening illness. It was disrespectful at best and inhumane at worst. Yet none of the representatives I spoke with took any interest in my situation. I could have been talking with someone offshore for all I knew. They simply said that as far as they could tell there was a problem with the billing codes. They did not know who made the mistakes, and I was responsible. If I did not get it straightened out, I would be responsible to pay the hospital bills directly. It did not matter to them that, within days, my physical condition would again be deteriorating to the point where I would not be in a position to handle the situation.

And you wonder why people are so frustrated with our health care system?

When the chamber's annual insurance renewal came, another company gave us a bid for our business, and we switched insurers to Blue Cross of California. I did not make the decision, but I am glad the change was made. Blue Cross has been an excellent example of how health coverage should work. I've had no problems or issues with the company, From the day coverage began Blue Cross assigned a case manager to me and that individual became familiar with all aspects of my claims. We have had no problems with Blue Cross and they have taken the position that their role is to pay legitimate claims, not to reject them.

Thank you, Blue Cross.

## Chemo Round 2

The week at home ended far too soon, actually sooner than planned. I was called back a day early for round 2 of chemo. They told me that this cycle would be easier. One of the chemo drugs would not be as strong, and another was equally as harsh, but they thought that I should be able to tolerate them adequately given my round 1 experience.

I wish it had turned out that way.

Throughout this time, I had my daily chores to do just to stay well. There was regular mouth care. That meant brushing my teeth, rinsing, and cleaning eight to ten times each day. I took special antibiotic medicines after each meal. We had to clean the catheter each day. Eating and sleeping were duties because they would contribute to my healing.

I had to concentrate on staying positive, being focused, and remaining optimistic. This was a full time job. There were so many things to do—even though I was weak and very ill. But my support group was solidly behind me.

I deliberately had few visitors in the hospital. Just getting into the BMT unit was a chore for visitors. First, visitors had to go through five minutes of hand washing. Next, they had to step on a glue mat that took contaminants off of their shoes. Then they went into the main nurse's station for gown, gloves, and mask. Then into the patient's room. It was quite the ordeal.

One regular visitor to the unit was Los Angeles cardinal Roger Mahony. We had worked together on some projects so we knew each other, and I was humbled by this Prince of the Church's desire to pray for me and with us. It was truly spiritual.

Because of the continual e-mail updates Karen sent to my list, it was easy for people to know how I was doing—and when things were not going so well. These e-mails generated so many cards and letters that we could barely keep up with them. I was heartened by the tremendous support I was receiving from friends and family. I could not have done it without them.

We hung every card or message I received on the walls of my room, and by round two it was filled with cards, letters, posters, and well wishes. After a short period of time, there was no more space on the walls. I received over one thousand such messages and cards. It was truly moving, humbling, and hard to believe.

One funny and rather humbling moment occurred. My job was very political and put me in contact with national and world leaders. I received notes from former president George H. W. Bush, former British prime minister Margaret Thatcher, former Canadian prime minister Brian Mulroney, General Colin Powell, and many others. But one day Pamela came home to this message on the answering machine:

"Hi Pamela and Rusty, this is [Senator] Bob Dole here in Washington. Rusty, I heard about your battle with cancer, and both Elizabeth and I wish you well. I don't have much to do these days and am good at running errands, so please feel free to give me a call if I can be of any help!"

What a surprise call! He was truly being kind, and we were so appreciative of him taking the time to call.

In this round of chemo, the doctors used a drug called high-dose Ara-C that, in a small fraction of patients, has side effects that can interfere with motor and neurological functions. If unchecked, these could be permanent.

In order to determine whether a patient is having these side effects, the nurses are required to administer various physical and mental assessments three times a day. These include asking questions, taking handwriting samples, etc. They told us about the risk associated with the drug, while at the same time advising us that this drug was a necessary part of my therapy. So we went forward.

I experienced the same results as I did in round 1 during the first week of round 2. Unfortunately, after a week, my legs went into spasm, and my handwriting became gradually illegible. They took me off the high-dose Ara-C immediately and substituted a lower dose of Ara-C.

But in the second round of chemo, I took a turn for the worse. While I experienced many of the same side effects as during round 1, they seemed to be magnified. The A-fib came back with a vengeance.

One story I will never forget occurred early one morning. I was having a severe A-fib episode—my heart rate went over two hundred beats per minute. The nurses called Dr. Douer (he is the head of the BMT department at USC and was on service that morning). Dr. Douer, a world renowned physician in this area, came in with a group of fellows and residents. The new doctors began talking about options for regulating my heartbeat; they talked about cardioversion, drugs, injections, etc. On the other hand, Dr. Douer looked at the heart monitor, sat at the edge of the bed, and took my hand. He talked to me calmly for several minutes and, as he was doing that the other doctors were transfixed on the heart monitor. The more we talked, the calmer I got, and within minutes his medicine of compassion and calm settled my heart and brought the A-fib under control. The new doctors were amazed and, at the same time, we all learned a valuable lesson; sometimes the best medicine is patience, a calm hand, and a warm heart.

Then within days, came a new complication—septic shock.

Septic shock is a serious condition that occurs when an overwhelming infection leads to low blood pressure and low blood flow. Vital organs, such as the brain, heart, kidneys, and liver may not function properly or may fail. Septic shock can begin with a fungal infection as it did in my case (rarely from a viral infection), or can be the result of various risk factors such as a major underlying illness, the leading one being hematological cancers, with leukemia leading the way. Unfortunately, I had both.

Once septic shock sets in, the patient is in an acute medical emergency and usually winds up in intensive care, which I did several times. The shock to the system is critical and often results in high or very low temperature, chills, shortness of breath, rapid heart rate, and variations in blood pressure. I had them all.

My septic shock was complicated by the congestive heart failure and A-fib because my heart was just not strong enough to fight back. Congestive heart failure results from the heart not pumping efficiently enough to the point where fluid builds up around and overloads the heart.

But somehow I made it through three episodes of this life-threatening complication as well. I would only learn later how dangerous it was—and that Pamela and the doctors talked about the fact that I might not survive it on top of suffering from the A-fib and rebounding from the other complications with which we were dealing.

I continued to do my best to keep up at work, doing all that I could to talk with the staff and management team as often as possible. I wrote my weekly column and participated in developing our business plan for 2004. I spoke and discussed strategy with the team. I was convinced that it was just a matter of time before I would be back at my desk doing the work I loved. And, it was an important part of keeping me engaged and not allowing my mind to wander to my problems. Without Marlee, David, and the rest of the team, it would not have worked; they were of great support.

After six weeks in the hospital, I was sent home to rest before round 3. But it would only be three days before I was summoned to return. I had the same routine at home as after round 1 although I was noticeably weaker. And, by this time, not only was all my hair gone, so were twenty pounds.

## Chemo Round 3

The ride back to Norris was very emotional. I knew that I was again leaving the family, but this time the streets glistened with the decorations of the holidays. Thanksgiving would soon be here, followed by Christmas, Hanukkah, and the New Year. The kids would be having their birthday in late November. Would I be in the hospital during this time of year? Would I have an easier time in round 3? It wouldn't take long to find out.

By this time, I had become even more aware of the predicament I was in. I had now spent most of the last several months in the hospital—something I never imagined I could do. I was without much contact with my children and my wife for most of this time. I was isolated and alone. To understand how isolating it is, just think of being alone in a room most of the time, interrupted only by occasional visits from doctors and nurses. And when your loved ones come to see you they are dressed in gowns, masks, and gloves. Perhaps your spouse could lay in the bed with you and you could hug for some minutes, but you could share no intimacy, much less closeness. Interactions that are meaningful, funny, and trivial are nonexistent. The nights grow long. The days are boring. The worry about family is endless. The ability to concentrate on things large and small is diminished.

But I knew that I had to endure and show courage in order to survive.

Thanksgiving was approaching and, once again, my health began to deteriorate. The chemo was still bringing harsh results to all parts of my body, and I was beginning to grow tired and weary of the symptoms. By now I had lost nearly all of my dignity and shyness as well as any self-consciousness I ever had about myself, my body—indeed, about my being. I allowed the nurses to do anything and everything they needed to do without protest or embarrassment.

Time, under these circumstances, was endless. Time in my room, alone, staring at the walls. Time in the hallways, on a gurney, waiting for a test to be taken or waiting for a doctor to talk about the latest test results. Endless time to think, contemplate, and to ponder. It plays games with you because you just cannot escape the bonds of time.

The week before Thanksgiving, I experienced the first of what would grow to become an ongoing problem that plagues me to this day.

I was feeling stronger than normal and decided that I would surprise Pamela and take a shower. In the past, she always helped me and got herself as wet as I did, although she was fully clothed. I wanted to do it myself so she could see that I was making progress. I consulted with the nurses, and they approved after watching me get out of bed and ambulate. They agreed to stay with me and help if I needed it.

Step one was to utilize the bathroom. After taking care of business, the next thing I knew I was on the floor, having fainted and banged my head on the tile walls. The nurse outside the room did not hear anything nor sense that anything was wrong until I pulled the emergency rope. Within seconds, five nurses were there. As I lay there half dressed, they formed a human stretcher with their arms and lifted me back into bed.

If you have never fainted, it is a scary thing. Whether you black out or not, you have the sensation of falling—and you don't know why. You try and grab on to anything that is near and can't do it because you either miss or just don't have the strength. It is a helpless feeling. Fortunately, all I came away with this time was a small bump on the head. But there were changes coming.

I was allowed no more unsupervised showers. I was confined to my bed, and a bedside commode would be my partner for days to come until my doctors were convinced I was stable.

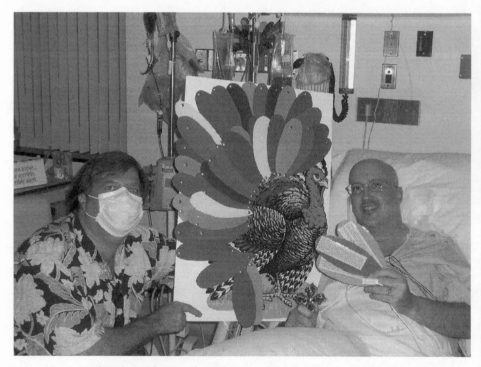

Rusty and Steve with Karen's creative turkey and inspirational messages.

The following week brought Thanksgiving and yet another crisis.

One of the first surprises was that Steve, Karen, and Sam came down for the holiday. Karen brought with her one of the many creations she conceived to keep my spirits up. It was a cardboard turkey with feathers that counted down the days to Thanksgiving. Each day had some type of motivational or spiritual message or notes from friends. I looked forward to reading them every day.

Her messages were accompanied by little gifts:

- A penny to remind you that you are very lucky
- A mint to remind you that you are worth a mint
- A rubber band to remind you to be flexible
- An angel to be your guardian and protect you

These were not the only such creations. She did the same thing at Christmas or for no particular reason at all. Karen was always thinking about things to take my mind off the treatments and pain and give me reasons to be hopeful and optimistic.

Karen was of tremendous assistance to us during this period, actually throughout our entire journey. At this point in the process, she and Pamela began to research the options we would have in the future, specifically should the need arise for me to have a bone marrow transplant. They made a direct outreach to the staff at Norris who put them on hold, much to their surprise and dismay. By this point in the chemotherapy process, I still had active leukemia; I was not in remission. So why wait? Why should we not move forward and see whether my brothers were a match or whether there was a match available through the National Marrow Donor Program?

The staff said that there was plenty of time to look at that in the future, but we just could not wait. The two of them researched transplant centers and collected all of the information they could on the transplant process. We talked about moving to the next step on the transplant road; however, the staff at Norris did not want to engage until they were certain I needed a transplant. It gave us great concern because we did not want to wait until the last minute to get started. But we were the amateurs, and they were the professionals, so we went along—somewhat blindly.

Having been in the BMT unit for most of the last few months we came to know the other patients. One such patient, Bill (an alias), had an autologous transplant (in which a patient's own cells or tissues are removed for later transplant back into the patient) because a suitable donor had not yet been identified. It was a stopgap measure to buy him more time.

Bill's devoted wife came to see him every day, despite the fact that she had to drive sixty miles each way after a hard day as a school principal. We were so fortunate that Pamela was not working outside the home. That allowed her to focus her time and energy on me and the issues relating to my wellness. I can't imagine the added burden if she'd had to drive so far each day. She brought food and stayed most of the evenings and on weekends.

Bill and his wife and Pamela and I decided that it would be fun to have Thanksgiving dinner together. Our families made dinner with all of the Thanksgiving trimmings and shared it with the nurses and staff in the BMT unit. Despite not being hungry or able to eat much, I managed a piece of turkey and even got out of bed into a wheelchair to share a few moments with the nurses as we dined together. Bill and I both had to stay in our rooms, but the nurses allowed us to open the doors so we could talk to each other and to the families and staff that gathered around the nurses' station. I even managed to offer a toast to all of us. But by later that evening, my world again began to collapse.

One of the dangers to people undergoing the type of rigorous chemotherapy I was subjected to is the possibility of infection. Patients with suppressed immune systems are particularly vulnerable to infections. That is why the rooms we live in have pressurized air, which means that air blows in the room at a greater rate than that outside the room. Therefore, when a door is opened, the air pressure blows air and contaminants outside of the room and prevents them from coming in the room. In theory it works and is yet another safeguard against infections. But that, even in combination with gowns, masks, and gloves is not always enough. We learned that the hard way. I managed to get yet another infection.

The infection came on quickly in just a few hours on Thanksgiving evening and manifested itself in a high temperature at first. Then I became lethargic, and all of the classic signs of an infection set in. But it moved so quickly that it was diagnosed as another episode of septic shock.

Once again I went into congestive heart failure and respiratory distress. I became delirious, and, by midevening, I was semiconscious. Pamela was told that it would be touch and go. If the doctors could not get the infection under control, the outcome could not be predicted.

I have never been one who believed in miracles. The mysticism of it all is puzzling, and, before that evening, I don't even know whether I would have recognized one. But that evening something happened that I now view as a miracle.

At some point that evening, when I didn't even know how close to death I was, I had a clear vision of my deceased parents. I vividly recall hearing their voices. They told me that they were with me and that I should hold on to life with every ounce of breath and strength I could muster.

Soon thereafter I heard another voice, but I did not see a vision. He identified himself as Jerry, Pamela's brother who was taken by leukemia as a teenager. He told me that everything was going to be OK.

There were no bright lights, no strange images. All I saw or heard were the visions and words of people who soothed me and gave me the courage and the will to get through the night.

Was it a dream?

Was it a miracle?

I didn't know and didn't care. I had never had such a vision and frankly had been skeptical when people told me that they had them. But to me this was clear as a bell; I will never be a doubter again.

By the next morning, I turned the corner. My temperature broke, and another crisis was over—for now. But it would not be the last episode of septic shock.

Two things happened that evening that I don't remember, which were told to me some time later.

I had a male nurse on my team that evening. He had worked with me many times before, and we had a great relationship. Apparently, while I was delirious, I called him over to ask him a question, and when he came to my bedside I put my arm around him and called him "Sweetie." The room burst into laughter. I don't remember a thing! Even if I remembered it, I probably wouldn't admit it.

Later that evening, in the midst of the crisis, I called Sam over to my bedside and asked him, in a quiet whisper, what kind of "pie" Gerald wanted for Christmas. I was sure I asked him what type of snowboard Gerald wanted, but everyone in the room stood by

Sam's story. It was the second laugh they had at my expense that evening. At least they had something to laugh at.

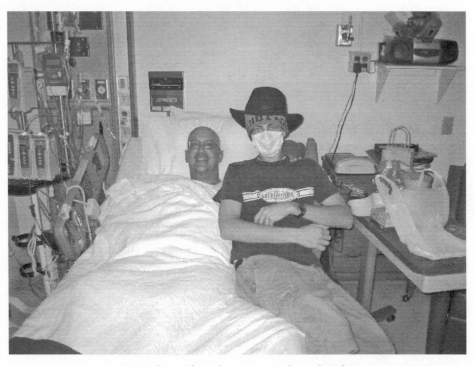

Sam always found a way to make us laugh.

By the weekend, I was myself again. The antibiotics, countless transfusions, and intravenous feeding brought my strength back quickly. I would spend the next three weeks at Norris, recovering from the complications and side effects so that I would be strong enough to go home and spend the rest of the holiday season with my family.

Up to this point I had been through three rounds of chemotherapy, and there was no sign that the endless ticking of the clock was on our side. Yet only another bone marrow biopsy would tell.

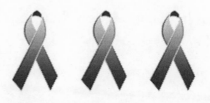

# CHAPTER 3

# THE POINT OF NO RETURN

*Only Time*[14]

Who can say where the road goes?
Who knows? Only time.
Enya

We now faced the toughest of choices—ones that would determine my ultimate survival: What were transplant options? Would we take the chance of destroying my immune system and taking the chance on a transplant in the hopes that I would receive a new one that would graft? What about an autologous transplant? What about no transplant at all and just stopping after chemo and radiation? Surely I would get into remission at some point short of a transplant and its enormous risk and danger, although the transplant would give me the best chance for long-term survival.

Difficult decisions. No easy answers.

---

14   http://www.lyrics007.com/Enya%20Lyrics/Only%20Time%20Lyrics.html

At the end of the day, there would be no guarantees; only time would tell.

At this point in my treatment, it really was the point of no return because the choices we made would put us on a path that would have a tragic outcome if the transplant did not engraft. Sure we could possibly obtain a second transplant and see if that worked, but that would be equally risky and would have long odds. Therefore, at this point, it was only time that would tell the outcome—time, that is, and modern medical technology and the skills of the doctors, nurses, and those who would care for me in the ensuing days, weeks, and months.

Just as I was recovering from the third round of chemotherapy, we received yet another serious blow. Dr. Khan gave us the news that the most recent bone marrow biopsy had revealed, somewhat unexpectedly, that the third round of chemotherapy had not put me into remission. In most cases, the chemotherapy does the trick, and radiation is the insurance policy. Transplants are then used for the toughest of cases. However, since the three rounds of chemo had not put me into remission, I would need the radiation treatments not just as an added measure, and I would definitely need a transplant.

I had to prepare myself for the worst combination of treatments you could ever imagine. It would be a harrowing experience, fraught with danger. It would take me down to the bridge of death, and then hopefully, my doctors would be able to bring me back to life.

To begin with, I would be bombarded with radiation. Following the radiation, I would receive additional lethal doses of chemotherapy to kill anything the first rounds of chemo and the radiation may have missed. That combination would destroy my entire immune system. At that point, I would be given a new immune system, either my own that will have been cleaned through an autologous transplant or one from a donor through an allogeneic transplant.

But that is not the end of it, because unforeseen complications or something called graft-versus-host disease (GVH or GVHD) lurks out there around the corner, which can be lethal or disabling as well. There is absolutely no way to prepare for the nausea, diarrhea, fevers, chills, sleeplessness, pain, etc., that you will experience, and, ultimately, the transplant might not graft, resulting in a tragic outcome.

However, we had the ultimate call on the transplant. I could opt to stop treatment with the last chemotherapy and take my chances. I could go on to radiation and see whether we achieved a remission—and take my chances. Or, I could go all of the way and take my chances with the transplant—the ultimate risk.

These are difficult choices, but we would soon learn that there were more hard choices ahead.

We knew that, having reached this point, there was no reason not to give medicine the best it had to offer me, so we decided that we would take the risk of the transplant. It was not a hard decision at the end of the day; if we did not go in that direction, I would surely not survive.

So here we were, nearly a month after Pamela and Karen first wanted to engage the Norris staff in discussions about a transplant, and now, in our minds, we had wasted time in the process of getting started along the road to preparing for a transplant. But it was what it was—and now the work to find a lifesaver for me would begin.

Once we decided that we would move forward with the transplant, the wheels were put into motion. Little did we know that in several homes around the country, people were being contacted because, at some time in the past, they registered with the National Marrow Donor Program (NMDP) to become a transplant donor for someone in need of a lifesaving bone marrow or stem-cell transplant.

A matched unrelated donor (MUD) transplant is the type of transplant that is least likely to result in a good outcome, and it is the toughest one for the patient because, unlike in autologous transplants or transplants from related siblings, in allogeneic transplants, the patient receives a completely foreign immune system.

The rules of the NMDP prohibit the disclosure of the name of the donor to the recipient or vice versa for one year following the transplant. This is done to preclude the donor from feeling guilty or taking on blame if the transplant does not result in a positive outcome, and it prevents the recipient's family from blaming the donor in the same event. I think it is a good rule. I know a donor whose recipient died seven months after the transplant and, while pained by her loss, I know that it would have been much harder on him if they had met.

Therefore, I knew almost nothing about my possible donor and would not for some time to come.

It was beginning to get more real each and every day. Since the chemo had not worked as expected, I would need the more extensive treatment and would be off work longer than expected. I contacted my executive committee and gave them the news. They were extremely understanding and committed to me that my job would be there when I was ready to return.

Despite the fact that Marlee had told me that she was planning to leave the chamber in early 2004 to be with her fiancée in New York, she stepped up to the plate, as usual. Knowing that the next phase of treatment would take several more months, she put her life on hold for me and said she would stay.

At this time, we knew little about transplants, but we soon received a graduate degree. We received most of our information from the NMDP, the national clearinghouse for allogeneic transplants. Information about the NMDP, which is a tremendous resource, is contained in the Appendix E.

A transplant, especially one from an unrelated donor, is a strong and dangerous treatment with serious risks, so it is not applicable to all patients. But we learned that a bone marrow transplant offers a patient the best chance to go into remission and, while remission is not a cure, it means that the level of leukemia cells is below a detectable level to confirm an active case.

There are two types of transplants—autologous and allogeneic.

For autologous transplants, the patient's cells are collected once he or she is in remission (usually after the second round of chemo), frozen, and readied for transplant. Autologous transplants have serious risks, but the risks are greater with allogeneic transplants. However, a patient has a greater risk of relapse after an autologous transplant and a better chance of sustaining a long-term remission after an allogeneic transplant.

In the event an allogeneic transplant is determined to be necessary, the cells can be obtained from a donor in several ways. First, the donor can provide bone marrow, which is usually taken from the donor's hips. This requires that the donor undergo surgery for a marrow harvest in which punctures are made, usually in the hip bones, to extract the bone marrow. The donor usually has a three-to five-day recovery period.

A second option is to obtain stem cells from the donor's blood in what is called a peripheral blood stem cell transplant (PBSCT). The PBSCT is much easier on the donor and is as simple as giving a blood donation, except that it takes several hours. However, there is no pain or recovery period for the donor other than regaining his or her strength by eating high-protein foods.

The last option is to use umbilical cord blood that is collected from infants at birth. The cord blood is frozen for later use. Unfortunately, umbilical cord blood is not a good alternative for adults because a significant amount of cord blood is needed to obtain the cells.

Each method had its advantages and disadvantages, and we would soon be discussing our options with the doctors.

The doctors at USC Norris talked frankly with us about the best chances for my survival. They were clear that, given the acute nature of my disease and given that chemotherapy did not place me in remission, my best chances would rest with an allogeneic transplant. We first needed to determine the type of allogeneic transplant before settling on the source of the cells. The three types of allogeneic transplants are:

Syngeneic transplant, in which one twin donates to another. (I don't have a twin, so that was out.)

Family or sibling transplant, in which a brother or sister donates. (My parents were deceased, but we would test my brothers.)

Matched unrelated donor (MUD) transplant, in which an unrelated donor is found through the NMDP. Unfortunately, 70 percent of those needing transplants do not have a suitable family donor and need to rely on unrelated donors. These patients, such as me, rely on the NMDP registry, which contains access to more than six million volunteer donors and fifty thousand units of cord blood.[15]

The first step in the process was to analyze my DNA characteristics to determine potential candidates. To make this analysis, my doctors performed a procedure called human leukocyte antigen (HLA) testing.

HLAs are found in proteins and the immune system uses them to recognize which cells are a part of your body and which are not, including those in your blood and organs. In order to be a candidate for a donation, the donor cells must closely match the recipient's in the HLA matching. This reduces the risk that the patient's system will attack the new cells from the donation and cause a rejection of the transplant.

HLA antigens are inherited, meaning that the best chance of finding a match is with a brother or sister. Since you inherit half of your HLA antigens from your mother and half from your father, each brother and sister who has the same parents as you has a 25

---

15  http://www.marrow.org/PATIENT/Donor Select Tx Process/The Search Process/HLA Matching Finding the Best /index.html#basics: "HLA Matching Basics"

percent chance of matching you. It is unlikely that other family members will match you.[16]

A close match is important for two reasons. First, it promotes engraftment of the transplant so that you begin immediately making new cells that will fight infections. Second, it reduces the risk of GVHD, a condition in which the immune cells you receive from the transplant attack organs in your body.

There are many HLAs. Transplant doctors look at only a small number of them for matching donors to patients. Since you inherit equal antigens from both parents, they look at three from each, or a total of six antigens. For adult transplants, the NMDP requires a match of at least five of these six HLAs.[17]

Most transplant centers, including the City of Hope where I would receive my transplant, look at more than six HLAs to select a donor. In my case, it was a total of ten antigens, and they wanted to match at least nine.

Once my testing was completed, the testing began on my brothers since they were the most likely donors. Unfortunately, neither Mark nor Lee matched adequately in the first six antigens. One matched three and the other matched two. It was an extremely disappointing day when we learned the news because that meant I would need to go the rough road of the allogeneic, unrelated transplant. It would be a road that would be much more uncertain, much more risky.

16   Ibid.
17   http://www.marrow.org/PATIENT/Donor_Select_Tx_Process/The_Search_Process/HLA_Matching_Finding_the_Best_/index.html#basics: "HLA Matching Requirements"

We knew that we had few options left. First, we could conduct bone marrow drives in our community and we could also work through the NMDP. It was only prudent to do both.

Before I began this journey, I knew little about transplants except organ transplants. Organ transplants are well publicized, and drivers in many states can opt to note on their licenses that they wish to be donors. I consider myself an educated person, but I knew very little about bone marrow transplants. I wish I had, for if so, perhaps I might have been able to have been a donor.

There are more than six million people who have registered for the NMDP. However, this does not mean that these people are all eligible. Some may have passed the maximum age to donate. Others may have passed away since registering. A potential donor may have had intervening health issues that make him or her ineligible. Others simply may have changed their minds about becoming a donor.

No matter the reason, there simply are not enough donors. Too many people die each year because a donor cannot be found. Beyond that, potential recipients who are from minority groups have a special problem because the registry is underrepresented by minorities.

There is no need for this to be the case.

With few exceptions, organ donations require a tragedy to occur before a life is saved. That is not the case with marrow or stem cell donations. Nobody will die by being a bone marrow donor. (I suppose it is possible in the most extreme case that a donor giving bone marrow through a marrow harvest in surgery could have a rare surgical complication that could result in death, but that is the case in any surgical procedure). There generally is no pain in giving a stem cell donation. All that is required are simple blood tests initially and blood draws for the actual donation. In the case of a marrow harvest, a donor does need to undergo a surgical procedure that can cause pain for several days, but those donations are becoming fewer each day. And now, a cheek swab is all that is required to initiate the process of becoming a donor.

With all of the efforts to improve technology to help people with serious diseases to survive, we can make significant advances by increasing the number of people on the registry to help people with not only blood cancers but other forms of cancer as well. I know too many people who have died waiting for a donor. In this day and age, that simply does not have to happen.

I had worked for seven years in Sacramento, and once my many friends in the area learned that I would need a bone marrow transplant, they came together in the fall of 2003 to conduct a bone marrow drive. Being president and chief executive officer of the chamber of commerce is a high profile job, and I was widely known in the community. The drive caught the heart of the entire community because it was inspired by my mentor in Sacramento, Raymond Nelson and his wife, Marilyn. From the moment Raymond learned that I had leukemia, he was there by our side. Countless phone calls reassured me that I would be well and that he would be there for anything I needed. He made trips to Los Angeles. And, most importantly, he pledged his energies and resources to conduct the largest blood and bone marrow drive Sacramento had ever seen. The drive would be in my honor and would mobilize the community.

A very good friend, Tom Sullivan, who has the number-one daily radio talk show in the market, got behind the drive with great gusto, devoting a show to the drive and to the need for donors. Our very good friends Bernard Bowler and Doni Blumenstock, came to Raymond and Marilyn's aid behind the drive. They raised money from area hospitals and area companies that underwrote the blood draw and testing costs. They recruited the area blood supplier, Blood Source, who got behind the drive immediately. The drive attracted nearly one thousand people who donated blood and/ or signed up for the bone marrow registry. It was a huge success, and both Raymond and Marilyn continued to support me as the months and years passed. Sadly and unexpectedly, just as I released this book for printing, Raymond passed away. I loved him deeply and will never forget him.

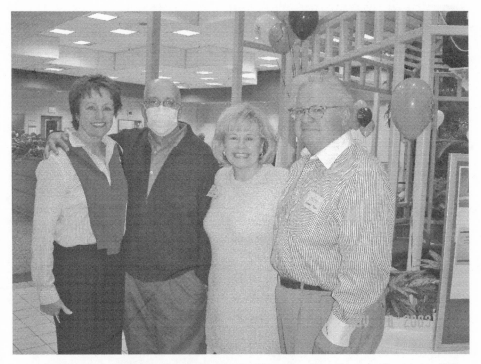

Pamela (l), along with Marilyn and Raymond Nelson, joined me at the Sacramento Blood and Bone Marrow Drive.

We made the flight from LA to Sacramento for the Sacramento Blood and Bone Marrow Drive. It was my first trip away from home since my treatment began. I was barely able to walk, but the energy Pamela and I received from these old friends lifted us tremendously. It was a humbling experience, seeing all of those people, many who did not know me, standing in line with their arms ready to be poked, hoping to save someone's life.

Smaller donor drives were conducted for me at a Los Angeles business owned by one of my board members, Ivan Nikkhoo; at the chamber headquarters; and in San Diego, which was run by my step-sister-in-law, Nancy Baum, and her family. Pamela attended these for me as I was too ill to join in.

These drives were of great comfort regardless of whether we identified a donor for me because we surely would identify a donor for someone else. One specific and instant outcome of the LA drive was that a donor was immediately typed and called to donate for a dying teenage girl. In fact, we now know of five people who became donors for other patients over the last three years! That alone, no matter whether I received a donor—or even whether I survived—allowed me to be at peace knowing that my disease had given the gift of life to others.

Beginning in early December, we began to focus on the transplant process. Since my brothers had not matched me, the doctors at USC recommended that we identify another transplant center, as USC did not specialize in unrelated allogeneic transplants.

We first consulted the NMDP's transplant center registry, which provided information on all transplant facilities in the country. The handbook listed each facility, the number of transplants it had made by type of disease, the facility's mortality rate, and a variety of other factors. It is an indispensable tool.

After reviewing the information, we decided that we would visit the City of Hope, located just outside of Los Angeles. The City of Hope had performed nearly eight thousand transplants, was the third facility in the country to do bone marrow transplants, and has a high success rate with AML patients. There were other options in Southern California, but we decided that we should start with the City of Hope. We considered other California locations in Sacramento and near San Jose (both places where we had friends and family), but the thought of moving temporarily on top of everything else was just too much to handle.

I did not know it at the time, but Pamela talked with Dr. Khan to discuss the reality of my present condition. She needed to know my realistic prognosis.

Dr. Khan sat her down and said that he was extremely concerned about my ability to survive for several reasons. First, I still had way too many leukemia cells after such harsh treatment, and perhaps they simply would not be killed fast enough to save my life. Second, he was extremely concerned that my weakened organs, having survived A-fib, typhlitis, septic shock, respiratory shock, and other conditions would not be strong enough to sustain my life. Only time would tell. Pamela would carry the burden of this prognosis silently on her shoulders in the months ahead.

That is not to say that I was not aware that my situation was extremely precarious. You cannot live from day to day with the ups and downs I experienced without knowing the severity of things. But when you are in the thick of things yourself, there is a certain sense of denial. Nobody sat me down and told me how things really were. Nobody actually said that my survival was in question. But I sensed that unless I applied everything I had to surviving, I might not.

We were blessed that a facility like the City of Hope was within driving distance. We have since learned that most transplant patients are not as fortunate. Most have to travel great distances and stay for months in a hotel or temporary apartments, away from friends and family.

Pamela and Karen made the first trip to the City of Hope to get oriented to the facility. They were impressed by the facilities and by the people they met. It is a National Cancer Institute-designated Comprehensive Cancer Center, and a research facility as well, that provides state-of-the-art care. Pamela and Karen were convinced that it was the right facility for us.

I was discharged from Norris ten days before Christmas, and the first order of business, despite my weakened condition, was to visit and receive a personal tour of the City of Hope. The City of Hope has a much larger BMT unit, many more services, and more experience than most other hospitals. Furthermore it specializes in unrelated donor transplants, the type I would be facing. Although its size did not provide the same intimacy as did Norris, we received excellent care from the doctors, nurses, and specialist on our team. Its reputation as one of the country's leading cancer and transplant centers is well deserved.

Dr. Anthony Stein, who would be my hematologist and be responsible for my care, gave me the tour. We got along well. He made us feel good about the staff and the facility's record of success, and, regardless of my concerns, I knew that the City of Hope was the best choice. The other facilities in the LA area did not have its history of doing unrelated transplants for AML in large numbers, and going away would be too much of a hardship on everyone.

Just days before Christmas 2003, we learned that the NMDP had identified three perfect matches for the first six criteria. Additional testing would need to be done, but we were heartened by the fact that there were donors that might be suitable for me. All too often, victims of leukemia do not live long enough to find a donor. The news that there were potential donors for me made the holiday that much more joyous. It was truly the answer to our prayers, and it gave us hope that I would survive. But we still had to wait—again. The NMDP needed to confirm that the donors were still willing and able to donate. In one of those homes, a family member turned out to have a DNA that was a close match to mine, and that family of three responded enthusiastically to being a donor if the match with me was determined to fit.

Although I would not learn the identity of my donor for over a year, I will now introduce him to you as Andrew. His wife's name was Sherry, and his son's, Alexander.

Even though Andrew was registered, he still needed to be tested to make sure he had not acquired infections or other diseases since he'd first signed up with the NMDP. The doctors at the transplant facility on Andrew's end had to ascertain that Andrew was still a qualified donor according to their standards, and he still had to give his final consent. Fortunately, all of that went well.

By the first of the year, we learned that the doctors had identified the donor they preferred: a ten for ten match, and he was willing and able to donate. Andrew, Sherry, and Alexander (although we still did not know who they were, or their names for that matter) would be a part of our family from now on, assuming things went well in the months to come.

Another blessing.

After the tour, Dr. Stein told us that the pathologists at the City of Hope had reviewed the USC pathology and confirmed the diagnosis—and also the fact that I was not in remission. The next step was to settle on the balance of my treatment.

We discussed many options including stopping at radiation and seeing whether I achieved remission, doing more chemo, or moving straight to a transplant. We had to keep in mind that my heart function was decreased and, because of the A-fib, I would not be able to survive total body irradiation (TBI). The alternative, spot radiation, carried with it the risk that the cancer would not go into remission prior to the transplant. So the choice of stopping at radiation was not viable because I could not get high enough doses. Secondly, since chemo alone had not worked so far, it probably wouldn't do the trick alone. We would just have to take our chances and take more direct radiation and hope that the spot radiation would kill the tumors and that there were not others lurking out there that they did not miss.

So, with the advice of the doctors, I was scheduled to undergo a three-week course of radiation that was targeted to the four tumor sites. I was never a fan of body piercing or tattoos, and I had told my kids so. It was therefore funny that I had to get tattoos for the radiation. These tattoos were placed on my body to triangulate the tumors and help the radiologists accurately aim the radiation. I wanted something fancier, like hammers or nails due to my name, but all I received were dots and arrows. How boring.

The radiation had its effects. Skin burns, mouth sores, nausea, and vomiting were the rules of the day. Fortunately, I did not have to be in the hospital for the radiation. I was allowed to go home each day. It amounted to three weeks of semi-normality, as the new normal was defined.

To keep things light, on the first day of radiation, I smuggled a set of plastic monster teeth in my clothes. After the first treatment and before the technician came back in the room, I put the teeth in my mouth. When she asked how I was feeling I opened my mouth with what looked like half of my teeth and said, "Well, I think it is OK, but I may have taken too much radiation!" We both laughed and became good friends.

Midway through the radiation treatment Dr. Stein, Pamela, and I discussed whether I should receive a marrow or a stem cell transplant. As I described earlier, the marrow is harder on the donor as it requires surgery whereas the stem cell transplant is essentially as easy as a blood transfusion. Dr. Stein recommended that I receive a stem cell transplant, which is known as a peripheral blood stem cell transplant (PBSCT). It would offer a greater chance for early engraftment and would be much easier on both the donor and on me. Upon Dr. Stein's recommendation, we agreed to proceed with the PBSCT.

After a happy holiday with friends and family, we received word that everything was set for the transplant, which was scheduled for January 21, 2004. Our prayers had been answered. There was an angel out there who would save my life.

Following the outpatient radiation and a series of other tests and doctor visits, I was admitted to the City of Hope in January and put on one final chemo regimen that would totally wipe out my immune system.

I was admitted to the City of Hope on January 11, 2004, which became day 11. They count down each day to day 0, which is transplant day. During those days, I received radiation and the final chemotherapy. After eleven days of treatment, I would reach that ultimate day, the day on which my transplant would take place.

Those eleven days were among the most difficult so far. The effects of the chemo seemed stronger because I was also simultaneously fighting the effects of the radiation. I reached neutropenia, with its effects as well. Overriding all of that was the knowledge that we were reaching the point where I would soon be at the true point of life and death. If things did not go well in the next few weeks, I would not recover.

The day arrived for Andrew as well, and, for him, it started off like any other, except that he would be saving the life of a perfect stranger.

On the morning of January 21, he drove the nearly one hundred miles to the nearest donor facility and began the two-hour process of giving his stem cells, after which they would be flown to California. As I described earlier, the process of making the donation is usually as easy as giving blood.

Usually, that is.

But things went terribly wrong. Malfunctions and other complications caused the nurses to tell Andrew, after nearly two hours, that it did not look like the donation could be successfully completed and that they would notify my transplant center that they would need to go to the next person on the list.

Andrew refused to accept that. He told them he had a deep feeling that I was in need of the transplant immediately and that he would be willing to do whatever was necessary, including undergoing the more difficult and painful surgical process of a marrow harvest if necessary to make sure I had the cells I needed.

Andrew insisted that they continue trying. The nurses kept on.

After ten more hours (twelve in all) and extremely uncomfortable consequences (for example, since he was not able to get out of the chair the entire time, he needed to be catheterized in order to urinate) they were able to obtain the cells they needed. It was off to the races in more ways than one. The cells were packed and rushed with a nurse to the airport for their lifesaving flight to California.

Little did Andrew or the nurses know, I was on day 0, and if I didn't receive the cells within twenty-four hours, I would be facing a difficult outcome.

Little did we know that back at the donor facility, one problem after the next had been putting my transplant, and my life, in jeopardy.

The tension was high as things were. We then received some unexpected news; the transplant would be delayed by a day. We assumed that the delay was due to transportation issues and had no idea of what had really gone on. We did not dwell on it, but we were concerned. We knew that I was in a precarious state, as are all patients on day 0. The fact of the matter is that the chemo and radiation are designed to kill your entire immune system. As a result, the body has no capability to fight infection or any outside influence.

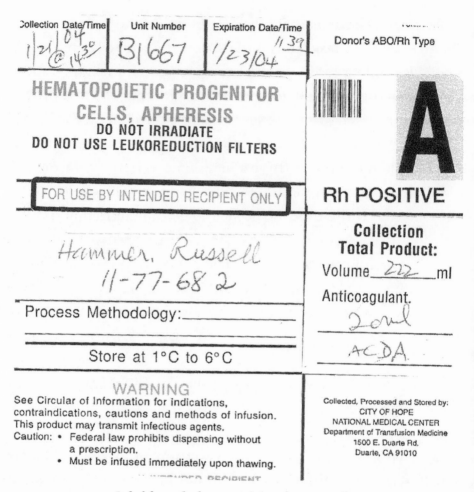

| Collection Date/Time | Unit Number | Expiration Date/Time | Donor's ABO/Rh Type |
|---|---|---|---|
| 1/21 04 @ 14³⁰ | B1667 | 1/23/04 11 39 | A |

**HEMATOPOIETIC PROGENITOR CELLS, APHERESIS**
**DO NOT IRRADIATE**
**DO NOT USE LEUKOREDUCTION FILTERS**

FOR USE BY INTENDED RECIPIENT ONLY

**Rh POSITIVE**

Hammer, Russell
11-77-68 2

Process Methodology:_____

Store at 1°C to 6°C

**Collection Total Product:**
Volume___222___ml
Anticoagulant.
2 oml
ACDA

**WARNING**
See Circular of Information for indications,
contraindications, cautions and methods of infusion.
This product may transmit infectious agents.
Caution: • Federal law prohibits dispensing without
a prescription.
• Must be infused immediately upon thawing.

Collected, Processed and Stored by:
CITY OF HOPE
NATIONAL MEDICAL CENTER
Department of Transfusion Medicine
1500 E. Duarte Rd.
Duarte, CA 91010

Label from the bag containing the stem cells.

And now we were in the third phase of my treatment, the most dangerous phase, when I would either get a new immune system or succumb to the lack of one. We had to have hope, for it was all we could hold on to. We had to have faith that the transplant would engraft and be successful. It was our only hope. We could not focus on the delay. One day should not make much of a difference, but it was unnerving.

I did not sleep at all that night.

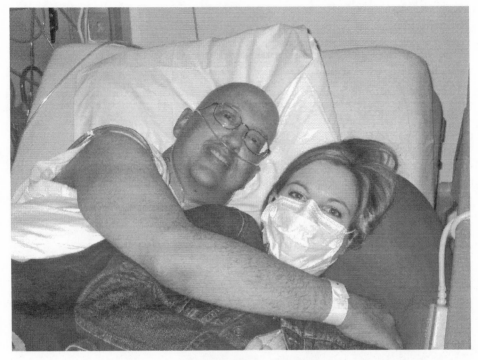

**Hugging Jennifer in bed.**

The next morning, we learned that the stem cells had arrived. The transplant would move forward. But not before we had completed a detailed preparation regimen of blood tests and pre-transplant medications. I was examined by several doctors, and Dr. Stein finally cleared me late in the morning.

Pamela and the kids were there early in the morning. They knew I was scared. I knew they were as well. I would soon be receiving a new immune system that we were counting on to save my life. It was as scary as a major transplant surgery, such as a heart transplant. However, if a heart transplant does not work, a patient can be kept alive on machinery until a new heart is found. In the case of a stem cell transplant, there are few alternatives. If the graft and your own system fight against each other, there is no other transplant immediately available.

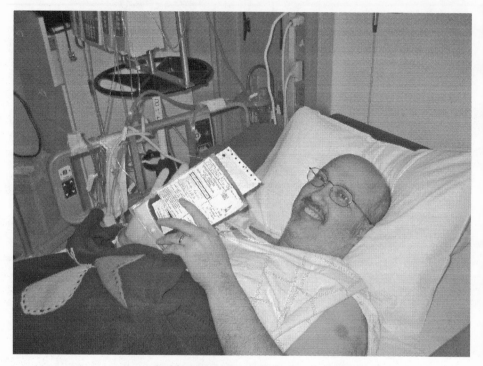

Rusty holding the stem cells before infusion.

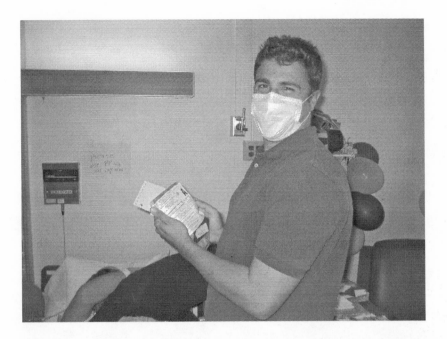

Gerald and Jennifer each hold the life saving stem cells before the transplant.

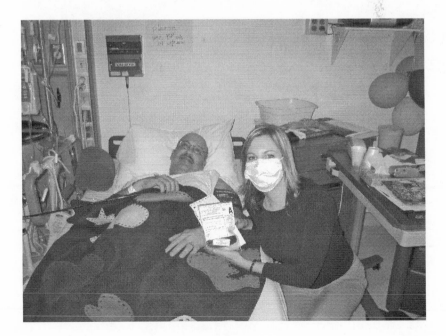

We talked that morning about our lives, our hopes, and our dreams. We cried and hugged each other. Pamela, Jennifer, and Gerald took turns lying in bed with me. There was fear in our eyes—fear of the unknown and the uncertain, but we had love for each other in our hearts. We knew it just had to work. We had done everything the doctors asked of us.

On Thursday, January 22, around noon, I managed a smiling game face amid the fatigue and pain when the nurses came in with the bag of stem cells that would save my life. It would be my new birthday—indeed hopefully the first day of the rest of my life.

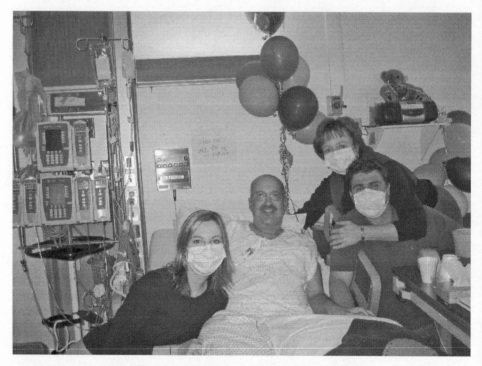

**We all gathered together prior to the transplant.**

The transplant itself was truly an uneventful procedure. In fact, it was probably the easiest thing I'd had to undergo. The two nurses came into the room and showed us the bag of blood that contained the lifesaving stem cells.

At first we could not believe that this simple bag contained the cells that would save my life. Pamela, Gerald, Jennifer, and I each held the bag for what seemed like an eternity. I never asked them what they were thinking or what they may have said to display their faith, confidence, and hope.

As for myself, I knew deep down inside that we were preparing for the moment of truth. Having survived the chemo and radiation, and now without an immune system, I knew what would happen if the transplant did not engraft. I simply and silently thanked all of those who had brought me this far; I asked that those who were caring for me be blessed for what they had done for me—and for what they would do to save my life in the weeks and months ahead. I thanked my then-nameless donor. I gave thanks for all of our friends and colleagues who were standing with me. I asked my parents and Pamela's brother, Jerry, to welcome me if things did not go well. And finally, I said my last words to Pamela, Gerald, and Jennifer. At that moment, as they introduced an entirely new set of immune cells—what is in essence an entirely new person—into me, I did not know I would ever wake up, or if I did, in what condition I would awaken or what my prognosis would be.

Then the moment arrived. The nurses hooked the bag of stem cells to my catheter and let it flow.

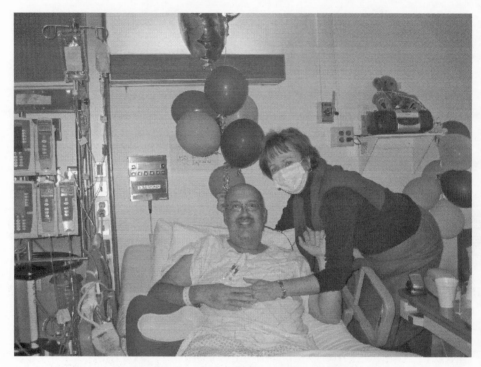

**One last hug before the transplant begins.**

It was totally surreal; it was almost as though we were in a new world. Here I was laying there on death's bed while we watched the possibility of new life flowing through a small tube into my veins. It was not cold; it was not warm. I felt absolutely nothing. The four of us then hugged and cried together, and I fell asleep as the life-saving cells trickled into my body and the waiting game began. In many ways, although the previous six months were extremely difficult, the real battle was just now beginning.

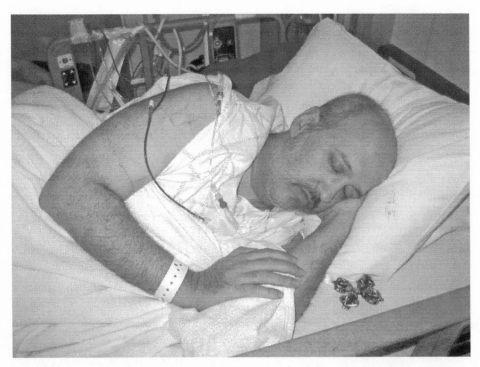

Once the transplant began, I fell asleep from exhaustion and allowed time, fate, faith, and modern medicine to take its course. The Dorje (see pg. 208) is at my side.

Here I was, at the virtual edge of death, yet with the possibility that new life was trickling into my body. We'd endured much on the road to this day. We knew the stakes. If the transplant engrafted, it could save my life—but there was no guarantee.

All we could do was to play the waiting game—again.

Those of you with leukemia are in a whole different universe. They treat you with chemo then take you down to near death and try to

bring you back to life. We work with it every day. We can empathize
with you but we can't even imagine what you go through.[18]
—Holly Gautier, director, Stanford Hospital
Cancer Concierge Program

The first three weeks following the transplant are the most risky
days of the entire process. The first risk is that of infection. I was
not spared.

The most important question was whether the transplant would
take. Think of it as grafting an orange tree to an apple tree. Both
are trees. Both are fruit trees at that. The question is whether the
two human trees, my donor's and mine, with much in common,
will engraft, and grow as one. That is the challenge. And it is a challenge on so many levels.

Think of it for a moment. The blood supplies nourishment to all
of our vital organs, which, in turn, give instructions to manage the
human body. In order to run this machine of ours, this machine
must be constantly in tune at the highest level, which is why even
the smallest of infections can set it off. Imagine what can happen if
mismatched blood, or elements of DNA within blood (such as the
antigens I talked about earlier), fight against other antigens already
in the patient; there would essentially be war inside on a massive
scale. That internal war would create a biological and systemic
havoc that would bring about a disaster that even the greatest doctors and today's twenty-first century technology could not defeat.

The battles began in my mouth almost immediately. The infections
were so severe that I was not able to eat for days and weeks on end.
I needed to be fed though an intravenous tube in order to keep my
nutrition levels to the point where I would not become dehydrated.

18   From a personal conversation

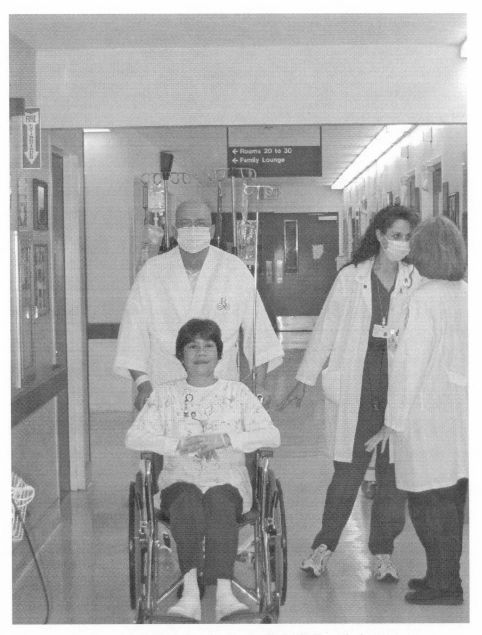

Occasionally I felt well enough to walk the halls with the nurses.
This day I felt well enough to push them.

Self-administered doses of morphine kept the pain under control—just barely.

In order to assure that the transplant engrafted, I was loaded up with antibiotics, antifungal medications, prednisone and a variety of other drugs to control inflammation, and antirejection drugs, some of which I take to this day and will for a long time to come.

Through most of these weeks, I was confined to bed. I would go many days unable to take a shower; it was lucky for the people around me that somebody invented premoistened body wipes. I don't have much memory of this time as I was weak, although I continued to remain in contact with my office and worked as much as I could manage.

One of the things that was most important to Pamela and I was to find ways to make some good out of my situation for other people. That opportunity came to us during this time period.

One member of the Los Angeles City Council, Jack Weiss, had been a stem cell donor in the recent past. He knew a lot about the problem of not having enough donors to meet the needs of patients. He came to us and asked if we would support a proposal to give any employee of the City of Los Angeles up to a week off with pay after making a donation. This would allow them to recuperate and not have to take time without pay for saving someone's life. We naturally agreed.

Pamela has been microphone and camera shy for most of her life, but when she feels strongly about something, watch out! She was called upon to be one of the featured speakers at the city council urging passage of Weiss's legislation. As a result of her heartfelt words and extreme passion for helping people afflicted with these deadly blood cancers, the proposal passed and opened up a very large donor pool for the NMDP. I was so proud of her!

Back at the City of Hope, the transplant grafted within forty days, but during that time, I continued to fight low blood counts and low platelets. I was accustomed to that from the chemo days. I was seldom strong enough to get out of bed. But I was making progress.

It was not an easy course, but my will and determination, the support of my family, and the great work of my medical team carried me through.

By the end of March, I was finally able to go home.

It was a welcome homecoming. The sights, sounds, and smells of the neighborhood were welcome. Just going in the house and seeing the furniture, photos, dogs, and keepsakes brought back memories that were only in my mind over the many months of absence. Although weak and tired, I did my best to get around the house and regain my strength. I had lost a considerable amount of weight and strength, but we were encouraged as I was able to walk around the house and even go outside from time to time. It seemed as though things were moving forward.

At this point, the burden of being my caregiver began to mount heavily on Pamela. The time in the hospital was tough; she had gone to the hospital every day, driving through heavy LA traffic, late nights, and uncertainty about my critical condition. But once I came home, the burden multiplied.

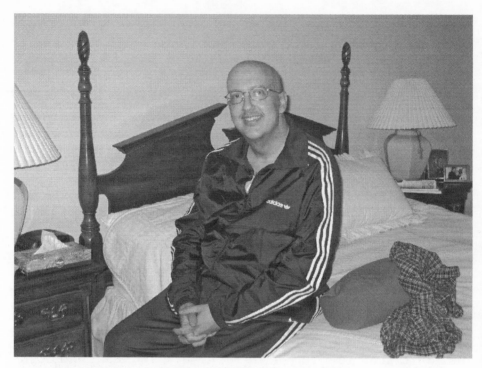

**My first day home after the transplant.**

There were medicines to administer (when I came home I was taking nearly fifty pills or other medications daily). Pamela made almost daily visits to the pharmacy. She had to drive me everywhere, especially back to the doctor several times a week. She prepared meals in accordance with the low microbial diet and continually did things for me that I could not do for myself. I watched with great emotional distress as she worked nonstop 24/7 to do anything and everything she could to make my reentry to home life as easy and comfortable as possible.

In addition to all of her home duties, she continued to work for the Majestic Foundation on its project helping inner-city youth and to assist the chamber by running our leadership development program when our executive director quit unexpectedly.

It pained me greatly to watch Pamela and others care for me. I had always looked out for my family, and the transition from being a provider to being totally dependent was an extremely difficult adjustment.

Beyond that, I became extremely distressed (and I supposed depressed as well) because my illness was sapping Pamela's life. She had come to LA hoping to resume her successful career, and now she was not able to do so. She simply placed me and my health above all else and could not engage in her career. In many ways, she began to lose herself as she became absorbed in caring for me. It has been truly heartbreaking for me to watch. Beyond that, it has been difficult for me, as someone who has always taken care of myself and my family to be forced to sit back and watch and be in a dependent role as others take care of me 24/7.

Within a short period of time, I began to regain more strength and feel better. I began to go outside more often, although I had to be careful with exposure to the sun due to my medications. I started to receive friends and colleagues we had discouraged from visiting at the hospitals. Coworkers came by, and we held meetings. It was beginning to be more like normal times again. I could see the light at the end of the tunnel. Little did I know that it was the light of an oncoming freight train.

On the inconvenient side, I had to wear a mask for the first one hundred days after I returned home whenever I ventured out of the house or had visitors. I could not be near young children or anyone who had received any live immunizations or were sick. I had to wash my hands constantly. Cleanliness was the order of the day. If we were not vigilant, my compromised immune system would not be able to fight off the effects of infections or viruses.

I learned immediately that two major things had changed. First, I was tired most of the time. The fatigue would force me to sleep in until 10:00 a.m., take a two- to three-hour nap, and be in bed by early evening. And, the more I tried to do, the more tired I became. I found that I could not see people for long periods. Meetings had to be kept to a minimum so that I did not get overtired. But at least it was progress.

Second, I found it difficult to achieve intimacy. I have since learned that one of the unspoken side effects of the treatment I underwent is a loss of interest, energy, and ability to be intimate. This has been a problem Pamela and I have been dealing with, and I am fortunate to have an understanding and loving mate who stands by me.

I could see myself getting better and gaining strength daily. Just meeting with people and being out of the hospital were tremendous victories. I was convinced that I would be back to work after a period of rest and recuperation at home.

Pamela had planned a campout for inner-city youth in the Malibu Mountains, which we both thought she should attend. It would give her some relief and the opportunity to get away from it all—if only for a weekend. The only way she would do it would be if someone was with me at the house all weekend, so a college friend, Sal, came down to LA and took charge. He did a great job by taking over and caring for my every need.

Up to this point, the treatment had generally gone along the lines we had expected, although it had taken a little longer. I was getting stronger. Most of the side effects I had suffered were predictable.

But by late April, just as things were looking up, we learned the hard way that things could turn on a dime. And we would learn that things were not under our control.

Several days after Pamela returned home from the youth campout, Karen was with us, and I awoke feeling extremely poorly. Pamela did not know what was wrong, nor did me, but I was dizzy, confused, weak, and delirious. I was on insulin at the time, the result of having contacted prednisone-induced diabetes, so the first thing we did was to test my glucose level.

Normal glucose levels are between seventy and one hundred twenty. That morning mine was at thirty, meaning that I was suffering from extreme hypoglycemia.

Hypoglycemia occurs when blood glucose level drops too low to provide enough energy. We would later learn that my level had dropped because I had been given the wrong directions for the amount of insulin to administer. Karen was with me as Pamela called the City of Hope and was told that I needed to get there as soon as possible. They carried me to the car because I was too weak to walk. Soon we were speeding toward the hospital, not knowing what was in store.

Dr. Stein and his staff immediately diagnosed me with diabetic shock and readmitted me. Despite the tension of the moment and its seriousness it brought yet another comical moment.

Upon being admitted to the urgent care unit at the City of Hope, I needed to get into a bed as soon as possible but was too weak to move. Pamela, Karen, and a nurse had the job of moving me from my wheelchair to a bed. But I had absolutely no strength to be of any help.

What happened next is somewhat of a mystery, except that the side effects were clear. The nurse, I am told, lifted me by the seat of my pants, off the ground and into bed. About thirty minutes later I regained my awareness and the first thing I discovered was that I was extremely sore in a certain area of my body, and I am told I shouted out, "Did someone grab me by the seat of my pants? My balls are killing me."

I am told that it was so loud that most everyone in the unit heard me and broke into uncontrolled laughter.

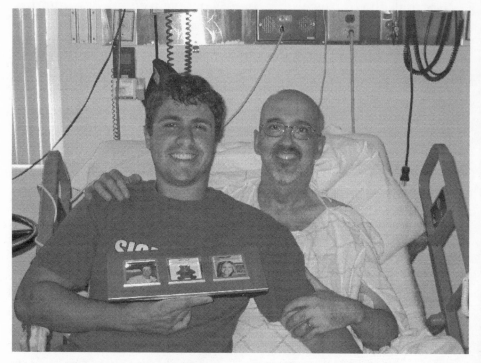

The seesaw of hospitalizations brought me back for my birthday.
Gerald is here with me.

I spent two weeks in the hospital, and then I was able to go home, but not for long. Over the next several months, I was in and out of the hospital more times than you can imagine. From bacterial to fungal infections, pneumonia to other issues, I would be in for a week or two at a time, then home, then back again. It was an absolute roller coaster, both physically and mentally. While we were prepared for some of the side effects, there was no way we were ready or conditioned for all that would come our way:

- My blood pressure would become highly unstable. As a result, I would be confined to bed because every time I would get out of bed I ran the risk of fainting as my blood pressure dropped—the result of orthostatic hypotension. Unfortunately, I would faint three times, with one of those spells resulting in a moderate concussion.

- I would contact two serious infections (cytomegalovirus and aspergillosis), which would cause a variety of unpleasant symptoms.

- I had yet another episode of septic shock that was as serious as the first one I had experienced at Norris.

- I would contact a staph infection that would begin in my central catheter. The infection would be extremely painful and not recognized initially by the doctors as an infection. It would be Pamela who correctly diagnosed it and who insisted on the blood cultures that confirmed it.

- We would never learn the reasons why, although it was probably a complication of the blood pressure, but I would develop severe varicose veins in my nose, which would bleed frequently. And when I say bleed, I mean it. For weeks at a time, I would awake to a pillowcase full of blood. It would get so bad that one doctor wanted to do surgery, which Pamela vetoed as being too risky. She was right, the bleeding ceased, and she saved me an unnecessary surgery.

- During one hospital stay, while my regular doctor was out of town for several days, I would begin looking at the trends of some of my blood work and would notice that my glucose levels had been running high for several days. The usual range is seventy to one hundred twenty, and I was running close to four hundred. Nobody noticed it, or if they did they did not talk with me about it. I would call it to their attention and would be informed that I probably had developed diabetes—but not to worry; it was induced by the high levels of prednisone and would "probably" go away. However, my mother had passed away from complications of the disease so I became concerned. Once they realized that I had "steroid-induced" diabetes, they would immediately place me on insulin to control my glucose levels.

- Some combination of chemotherapy and radiation had caused my production of testosterone to decline dramatically and it would not recover adequately on its own. One result was that I would begin to experience hot flashes that were not only uncomfortable but inconvenient. More drugs, which I must take most likely forever, would eventually get this problem under control.

- I would continue to have irregular and unpredictable episodes of atrial fibrillation.

- Once I had completed the transplant, the doctors became concerned that the leukemia may have crossed what is known as the "blood-brain barrier." If this had occurred, the leukemia could have penetrated the spinal column and gone to my brain, which would have been a serious complication. Rather than risk this, they'd ordered spinal injections of chemotherapy drugs that would occur weekly for six weeks. Believe me, spinal cord injections are nothing to dismiss; they are uncomfortable at best, and downright painful in most cases.

- I would have continual bouts with pneumonia.

- I would have bouts of graft-versus-host disease. During this battle between my body and the new immune system, wherein my organs attacked my new "foreign" cells, I would suffer a variety of afflictions. There is some good to having a little bit of GVHD; when treated successfully, it demonstrates that your body and your new immune system are working in harmony. GVHD mostly occurs in the liver, skin, and the GI tract. It can be either acute GVHD, which goes away after one hundred days, or chronic GVHD, which could last for years. Mine would be chronic GVHD—what else?

- GVHD would first show itself in my intestinal tract, which is one of the most common forms of GVHD. These bouts would cause severe stomach pain along with nausea, diarrhea, and other gastrointestinal distress. I would have two colonoscopies over five months; there is nothing more uncomfortable than a colonoscopy. Fortunately, the medications would bring the GVHD under control, although it is a condition that can reactivate itself at any time.

Treatment would take longer than any of us ever imagined: days, weeks, and months in the hospital. Lonely days stretched into wretched evenings. It was a terrible experience. All I wanted to do was to go home for good. I kept going back to the hospital over and over again. I am reminded of these days by the following words from the song.

*Home*[19]

Let me go home—I wanna go home
I feel just like I'm living someone else's life.
—Michael Bublé

Of course, my desire to go home was always strong. I spent so much time in hospitals that all I wanted to do was to go home. There were times when I thought that I would never be able to go home for good; that some day I would close my eyes in the hospital and never wake up.

I felt as though I was living another life—that my life had been cut down just when things were going right for us—but I knew just as well that we had to fight through all of the adversity if I had any chance of ever going home.

I continued to have significant problems with my heart. The hospitalization for that particular trouble lasted for about a month

---

19   http://www.lyricsdomain.com/13/michael_buble/home.html

and included several trips to the intensive care unit (ICU). The doctors determined that I needed to see a heart specialist, Dr. David Cannom, at the Good Samaritan Hospital in LA. Fortunately, in one of the rare instances where nothing was found that was serious, an angiogram determined that my arteries were clear and that I did not need bypass surgery. We would need to focus on treating the A-fib, but that was not a priority at this time given the other complications. In addition, dealing with the A-fib would require a surgical procedure for which I did not now have the strength.

After the stay at Good Samaritan, I was transported back to the City of Hope. The ambulance drivers set the gurney down in back of the ambulance—in the shining sun. It was the first sun I had felt on my face in months. I asked the drivers to just leave me there for a few minutes so I could soak up the sun. The warm breath of the sun on my face had never felt so good.

After a few more weeks in the hospital, I was allowed to go home and begin again to recover. Once home I started to get stronger and felt as though I was only weeks away from being able to go back to work on a part-time basis.

But things really broke down in July and seemingly, in retrospect, ran out of control.

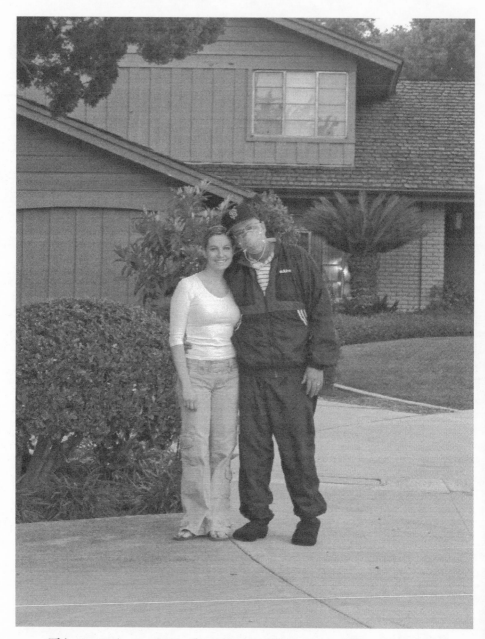

Things were improving in the summer of 2004. I was walking around the neighborhood with Jennifer the day before disaster struck and set me back in my recovery.

After taking a nap with Pamela on July 5, 2004, I got out of bed and took one step. The rest is fuzzy, but, to the best of my knowledge, I fainted (the result of problems my doctors were having in regulating my blood pressure). I fell softly on the carpet—only in the wrong way. Immediately, pain shot through my leg, I let out a deafening scream, and I could not move. Pamela knew that there was no way she could move me, and she also sensed that something was seriously wrong, so she called the paramedics. I had fallen between the television and chest of drawers with barely two inches on each side of my head. The paramedics arrived and examined me; they said that I had most likely broken my hip. We could not believe it.

The City of Hope is not an orthopedic hospital, so I was taken to yet another hospital. Once there the diagnosis was confirmed. I was in such pain that, over the next hour, I was given eighteen milligrams of morphine, an incredibly high dose in such a short period of time.

We did not know an orthopedic surgeon so we were assigned one at the hospital. Concurrently, Pamela called friends who gave her several referrals. The most revealing thing she heard, from one physician friend, was the name of one doctor he would not use. Coincidentally, this was the one to which we had been assigned.

Using her determination as a caregiver and her assertiveness, Pamela told the hospital that we would not accept this surgeon and proceeded to call in Dr. Norquist, who was recommended by our friend. Dr. Norquist came to visit me that Sunday night and determined that surgery would be necessary. However, I was so drugged that I would not become adequately lucid to have it for at least two days, given that this was not an "emergency."

After Pamela consulted Drs. Norquist and Stein, they decided that, while I probably needed a hip replacement, I would likely not be able to survive such an extensive surgery due to my low blood and platelet counts. As a result, the decision was to pin the femur so that I would spend a limited amount of time in surgery and reduce the risk of significant bleeding and other complications.

The surgery went well, but was just the beginning of yet another journey. I was placed in rehabilitation and physical therapy, but I was unable to walk without a walker.

The doctors suspected that something more was wrong and ordered a bone scan. The test revealed that I had contacted a severe case of osteoporosis—most likely the result of the high doses of prednisone I had been taking.

Osteoporosis is a disease in which the bones become extremely porous, are subject to fracture, and heal slowly. It often leads to fractures of the hip, spine, hands, and other bones.[20] It occurs especially in women following menopause (although the condition is occurring in men in growing numbers) and often leads to curvature of the spine from vertebral collapse.[21]

That reminds me of a funny story about the title of this book. I was developing conditions that are much more common in women (osteoporosis and hot flashes). One day, while talking with friends about this book, I proposed that the title should be *How I Became a Middle Aged Woman without Sex Change Surgery*. More people would probably be intrigued by the title, but the idea got laughter and went nowhere.

---

20   http://www.nof.org/osteoporosis/index.htm
21   http://www.niams.nih.gov/bone/hi/osteoporosis_men.htm

Three weeks later, I began to have severe back pain. When I went back to Dr. Norquist for an examination of the hip, I complained of the pain and he took some X-rays. He told me that I had sustained a compression fracture of two of my vertebrae as a result of the osteoporosis. For this, he ordered complete bed rest and confinement to a wheelchair.

Over the next few weeks, I sustained five more compression fractures, for a total of seven. I spent most of the next seven months in a wheelchair. I didn't realize at that time the extent to which this would set back my recovery. Not only was I fighting the complications of the treatment, I was now unable to walk or get any exercise which, resulted in a rapid deconditioning of my system. I lost muscle mass, strength, and stamina at an even greater rate. And my dependency increased by the day.

By the one-year anniversary of my diagnosis, I had spent 303 nights in the hospital.

In the summer of 2004, I developed a second severe case of GVHD, this one in the stomach that hospitalized me for seventy-three days. It was one of the most difficult hospitalizations of all because it came so unexpectedly and lasted for so long. But most of all, it marked the beginning of yet another major change in our lives.

It became clearer than ever that we were no longer in control of our lives. Hospitalizations occurred on a regular basis and without warning. Whenever I came home, I was optimistic, but unfortunately, my stays would seldom last for more than a few weeks, and I would be right back in the hospital. The uncertainty was maddening. Furthermore, the timing of my return to work was becoming less certain.

At home Pamela carried the complete burden on her shoulders. While Gerald and Jennifer spent some time helping her, she was truly on her own. We lived in a beautiful home in San Marino, which was near Pasadena. Keeping it in the immaculate condition it deserved was not easy. And the constant attention to my every need only amplified Pamela's stress.

If there was one thing that saved us emotionally during this time, it was our introduction to The Wellness Community. Founded in 1982 in Santa Monica by Dr. Harold Benjamin, The Wellness Community is an international nonprofit organization dedicated to providing support, education, and hope for people with cancer and their loved ones. Their counseling, support group, caregivers, and patient programs provided an oasis, specifically for Pamela, to talk with families having similar experiences. We have become so impressed by the Wellness Community programs that we are in the process of starting up a Wellness Community facility in Silicon Valley.

In late 2004, I was honored by the UCLA Bio Med, the research arm of the Harbor-UCLA Medical Center, at their annual Discovery Gala for my leadership in the region and for my courage in fighting leukemia. The formal dinner, in front of over five hundred of LA's elite, honored me as a cancer survivor. It was a great night—my first time in a tuxedo in a long time. I gave the first speech I had delivered in over a year; for someone like me who made speeches and presentations daily, it was an invigorating moment. I was back on the public stage again, albeit sick and not my former self. But I was there, and it gave me hope. We had a great time but paid in the currency of exhaustion. When we returned home, I could barely make it from the car into the house and was in bed for three days recovering. I prayed that this lack of stamina would not continue like this as it continued to point to my continuing fragility.

We decided that we needed to downsize by selling our home, which we did in the fall of 2004. Following a quick sale, we moved into an apartment in downtown Los Angeles, located only a few blocks from my office. It would be easier for Pamela and closer for me and my staff. It seemed like a good solution.

Our apartment would be our home through the middle of 2005. But over these many months, we learned why we didn't like apartment living. It was a small and confining atmosphere. Young people were everywhere, meaning noise at all hours. All of the inconveniences were there: garbage a hallway away, small appliances, a washing machine and dryer that could be heard throughout our small apartment, noisy neighbors always pounding on their floor/ our ceiling at night, mail in the basement, and someone periodically in our parking space. To make matters even more complicated, I was in a wheelchair the entire time making mobility that much more difficult. But without the wheelchair, I would be completely immobile. I therefore accepted it, but I hated every minute I had to sit in that iron prison.

Life in the apartment was difficult. I would have several more admissions to the City of Hope. There were countless clinic visits. It seemed like it was a never-ending parade. And the more I went into the hospital, the more difficult the stress of it all impacted Pamela.

The holiday season of 2004 brought some sad news to our family, but it was the type of news that we had grown to expect from time to time. Quite unexpectedly, a close friend and political mentor from Sacramento, Congressman Robert Matsui, had been diagnosed with what is called a myeloproliferative disorder. This disease is a forerunner of acute leukemia and, if undiagnosed, becomes full-blown leukemia. Bob had learned of his disease in late 2004, and he succumbed on New Year's Day to complications from his disease at the age of sixty-three. Unfortunately, his death had come so soon and suddenly that we had not had a chance to say good-bye.

Bob had been a charismatic leader, a politician beyond reproach, and a courageous and fine man. The country had lost yet another great leader to blood cancer.

Bob would be succeeded in Congress by his wife, Doris.

Throughout this ordeal, I remained president and chief executive officer of the LA chamber. The longer my illness dragged on, the more difficult things became. It was harder on me to keep up. It was tough on the staff because they could not talk with me as much as they would have wanted. And the leadership of the chamber, ever willing to work with me and support my return, was becoming concerned that I might never return. Once Marlee Miller left, as we had planned, I asked David Eads, who was our vice president of membership, to take over Marlee's place. He would do an outstanding job acting in my position, and I would promote him to the position of senior vice president. David would become a close confidant and would work with me in all areas managing the chamber and leading the chamber until my departure. Like Marlee, he stepped to the plate in ways I could not have imagined. I had a great team.

I do not want to be repetitive, but while I am talking about the staff, I must say that the entire group pitched in and did an excellent job while I was gone and the organization was leaderless. I do not use the word leaderless to take away anything from Marlee or David, but when an organization does not have a full-time president whose job is to provide leadership, vision, and inspiration to an organization, then something is missing. It is truly a tribute to the staff that they pulled together in my absence to show me what they could do and to how much they understood our mission and their roles, and to their capabilities. They truly excelled under the most difficult of circumstances and not only kept the organization but allowed us to keep the momentum moving forward along the growth curve we established.

In my absence, they did great work as individual contributors, as did a newly appointed CFO, Noly Lallana, and Brendan Huffman, who I selected as our new director of public policy, along with Marie Condron, our director of marketing and communications.

The more we talked, the more Pamela and I realized that the situation in the apartment was not working out. Even more important was that we had very little support locally to help us when I became ill or went into the hospital. The demands on Pamela did not let up; she was becoming exhausted and overwhelmed physically and emotionally. We talked about moving back temporarily to San Jose, where we had been raised. But we were stuck in the apartment until at least April 2005 because of our lease. So going to San Jose would not be possible until at least then.

A move to San Jose might be for a short period of time until I recovered, but it seemed like the only way that we could get the support we needed. I had lifelong friends still there. My brother and Pamela's brother, mother, and father were closer, as were many of Pamela's friends. While it would require transferring my medical care, it seemed that moving was the only way Pamela would get some relief, and it would give me the opportunity to be closer to people who could help me as well.

We really didn't know how we would accomplish this, as our income was somewhat limited at this point. I was on long-term disability; however, the policy had a provision that limited the amount I would receive, as the highest paid employee, to approximately 40 percent of what I had been earning. Therefore, we would have some limitations on what we could do.

Not really thinking how they would react, we talked with Karen and Steve about our options. We asked whether there was any way we could stay with them in San Jose for a short time. Within a nanosecond they said yes. We just could not believe it. It was the answer to our prayers and would aid in my recovery in ways we could not imagine.

We soon began making plans to spend time in San Jose, going back and forth. Gerald and Jennifer took a small amount of our furniture up one weekend in the fall and a week later Pamela and I drove up. When we arrived, I just could not believe it. Steve and Karen had completely rearranged their home. They had transformed their dining room into the family room and made the family room available to us. Our furniture fit perfectly. They had installed a wheelchair ramp at the front of their home.

They'd thought of everything!

It was ideal for us. When I went into the bedroom, it was the second time that I sat on a bed and cried, just as I had on the night of my admission to Norris. But this time I cried, not because it was small and unacceptable, like Norris, but because it was ideal and I was overcome with joy. That room became our home off and on through early 2005 and fulltime until August, 2005. I commuted for weeks at a time and was able to keep working part-time.

I cannot express the way we feel about Steve, Karen, and their son, Sam. They were there for us every step of my treatment. They traveled down to Los Angeles to help without being asked. They took the initiative to do anything and everything that was necessary. They took us into their home and allowed us to interrupt their lifestyle for nine months. They included us in their holidays, parties, and family gatherings. It was a show of love, loyalty, and commitment that is hard to find these days.

It was a rare situation. They are rare people. They were our angels.

We spent the holidays in San Jose and continued to commute back and forth. I went to the office as often as I could so that I could stay in touch with the staff, go through mail, attend meetings, and work on important meetings with the staff. I also attended a few board meetings. But as time went on I simply was not getting much better. I remained in the wheelchair most of the time. I could work from home and on e-mail, but I could not spend more than an hour or two in the office or at a meeting. I simply had to rely on others.

In January, 2005, I was able to attend the chamber's inaugural dinner for the first time since becoming ill. I was able to suit up in my tuxedo, rise from my chair, and give a ten-minute speech. Again, it was a great experience, and I received a standing ovation, but I paid for it for weeks to come. I once again found myself back in the hospital for overdoing it.

When would it end?

How would it end??

Would it ever end?

Work and recuperation continued through the spring, but I was in constant pain and made regular weekly visits to the doctor and occasional hospitalizations.

By the summer of 2005, I went down to LA and had dinner with the leadership of the chamber. I told them that we were spending time in San Jose to help with my recovery. They knew that we had sold our home and were concerned that this meant that I was leaving for good. I told them that was not the case; I just needed to get away to focus on my recovery, and I would continue to do the work I had been doing, just from San Jose.

We had previously set a goal that I would return in January or February 2006. It seemed reasonable at the time, and I was working at home and keeping up well enough. But I found that the fatigue and periodic hospitalizations were unpredictable. More than that, new side effects and complications seemed to come up without notice. It was now September of 2005 and, despite my emotional connection and my dedication to the chamber, I had to admit to myself that there was no way that I could accurately predict a date on which I would be able return. I had been back in the hospital too many times, and the admissions were unpredictable. Despite the fact that we were not only keeping things going with the chamber but, continuing to grow and command the respect and attention we deserved, I came to the conclusion that it was probably in the best interests of the chamber and my health that they begin to search for a successor.

There was a lot of gnashing of teeth that evening as we discussed our options. Deep down, I did not want to leave the chamber. I do not believe they wanted me to leave either. The relationship had been good for both the business and for me, and to have it cut short in this way was extremely disappointing for all of us. We had made so much progress in a relatively short time and there was so much more we could do together. But I thought I owed it to the organization to do what was best and I believe that, in the end, the board of directors appreciated that I essentially took the decision out of their hands.

They agreed, and that was that. We would announce it to the board later that month with the intention of having someone in place on March 1, 2006. As it turned out, it took until July, 2006. I kept working as president and CEO until that time and as a senior policy advisor for another eighteen months.

Below is the letter I sent to our members:

Dear Friends, Colleagues, and Members:

It is with both great optimism and heartfelt emotion that I write to inform you today of important changes within the Los Angeles Area Chamber of Commerce.

As some of you may already know, I have been engaged in a battle against leukemia and a variety of complications result-ing from this disease for some time. Your support and affec-tion for me and my family has helped carry us through these difficult times. Equally important has been the support of the Chamber's Board of Directors and leadership, under the chairmanship of George Kieffer and Chris Martin during this period. They have treated me with the respect and compassion that should serve as a model for all employers.

I have done my best over these many months to continue to lead the Los Angeles Area Chamber of Commerce as its president and chief executive officer. Through continuing to write the weekly Business Perspective, guiding our strategic direction, focusing on high priority projects, and continuing to build our Board and leadership, I have served the Chamber, its members, mission, employees, and our region to the best of my ability.

I had hoped that I would be able to return to work on a full time basis at the level of energy and commitment demanded of this position. However, the time required for a full recovery continues to be uncertain. For this reason, I have submitted my resignation as president and chief executive and have recommended that the Board begin a national search to recruit my successor. I have informed the Board of my decision, and they are proceeding based upon my recommendation. Until my successor is named, I will continue as president and chief executive officer serving the needs of the Chamber and our region, as I have since the day I arrived.

I was given the honor to lead the business community and the chamber of commerce in the second-largest city in America. During this period, the Chamber has enjoyed unprecedented growth and leadership. As a regional steward we have tackled the issues and challenges that will assure our future quality of life and economic prosperity.

Throughout my time in Los Angeles I have been blessed by many things; key among them have been the friendships that I know will last for years to come. While this decision is personally painful, I know it is in the best interests of the Chamber, me and my family. I would like to thank you for your ongoing support for me and my family, and for the Chamber, as we search for a successor to take the reins of this great organization. I will continue to be involved with the Chamber in the months ahead and look forward to working with you as my tenure comes to a close.

Sincerely,

*[signature]*

Russell J. "Rusty" Hammer
President and CEO

It was one of the most difficult things I have ever done. I loved the job. I loved the limelight. I loved being able to influence public policy at the highest levels in the second largest city in America. I loved the turnaround and the challenge of continuing to build the organization. I loved the people. We loved Los Angeles.

I tried as hard as I knew how to return to work. I went back to LA as often as I could, trying to work at the office and attend meetings. But the fatigue and difficulty of getting around was just too great. While at home or at the apartment, I could barely manage a few hours of work before succumbing to fatigue; yet I would work seven days a week. I would work all hours of the day, yet people did not always see it. I just could not do it. For now, my disease had temporarily derailed me.

The day I tendered my resignation was one of my lowest days since my illness was diagnosed. But having been a corporate CEO and a corporate board member I understood that the handwriting was on the wall and I knew what the board members were thinking. They would support me as long as I felt I could do the job, but they would leave that decision in my hands. It was up to me to make the right decision. I had to decide what was best for me and what was right for the chamber. And I knew deep down inside that the chamber needed me at the office and in public, every day talking to the community, working with businesses, dealing with politicians, and working with our opponents. I just could not do that and could not predict when I would be able to do so. Therefore, the right decision was for me to resign, despite the fact that I was never a quitter, and leaving was the last thing I would ever want to do. I never thought cancer, or anything like it would beat me. But for now, it had.

Thoughts swirled. Where would we live? What would I do for work? How would I support the family? Many questions. Few answers. And much like during my days in the hospital, I was not in control.

The family had discussed this subject several times, and they reassured me that my success and future was not defined only by the chamber. Despite the success there, they knew that I would rebound, in time, to redefine my life and my success at whatever level my health would allow. But for now, the important thing was to do what was best for my health. I knew they were right, and, as hard as it was, resigning was the right thing to do.

I was also comforted by hundreds of cards, letters, and e-mails from people congratulating me on the work I had done, expressing sorrow that I needed to retire from the chamber, and wishing us well. These messages were heartfelt, and they were extremely reassuring.

By the late summer of 2005, we had located a home in San Jose and moved there. Don't fool yourself; downsizing is not easy. People talk about it today as being the new thing in urban living—when you become the empty nester, you get rid of everything you don't need and can live in less space. Though perhaps true, to an extent, in reality it was tough. Try it some time.

San Jose is one of the priciest housing markets in the country, and moving back into it was not easy. That meant buying something much smaller, which would meet our needs. It also meant sorting through all of our furniture, papers, and personal items to get down to the bare essentials. It was not easy to do, and it was even more difficult given the fact that I could not participate. Pamela had to do it all, as she had been doing for the past few years.

After renting storage containers and donating furniture and other items, we were finally able to get all our remaining possessions in our cozy and comfortable downsized home.

Before moving to San Jose, I contacted a friend from my days in Sacramento, Martha Marsh. She had been president of the UC Davis Health Care System and was president of the Stanford Hospital and Medical Center. She helped me in the transition, and when we settled in, we transferred my medical care to Stanford under the

direction of Dr. Robert Negrin, the head of the facility's bone marrow transplant unit. It helps to know people in high places.

We could not have known at the time how well we would come
to know Dr. Negrin and the staff at Stanford.

Almost immediately, I was hospitalized for pneumonia. That
was followed by several more admissions through the end of 2005.

*The Godfather Part III:* [22]

Just when I thought that I was out, they pull me back in.
—Don Michael Corleone (played by Al Pacino)

One of those admissions was at about the same time as the
annual Leukemia & Lymphoma Society's Team in Training Nike
Women's Marathon in San Francisco. Jennifer had run in the event
a year earlier and Pamela was running this year. I was so proud of
her; she had trained hard for many months and was the leading
fund-raiser in northern California.

By race day, I was still in the hospital so Pamela went to the run
with Gerald and had a great time. Unfortunately, that afternoon,
I had a major A-fib attack. To add to the situation, this occurred
over a weekend when my normal doctors were not on service,
and the floor was populated mostly by residents. There is nothing
wrong with residents (they are doctors as well), but all too often I
have seen them become overzealous trying to impress fellows and
attending physicians.

---

22   http://www.imdb.com/title/tt0099674/quotes

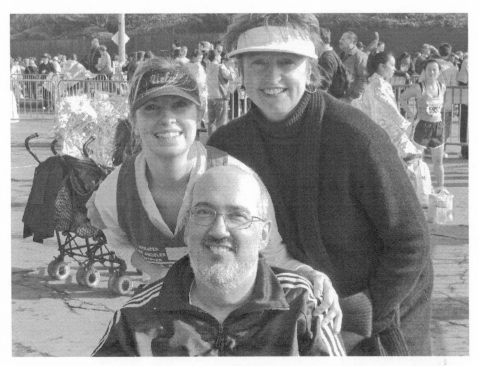

Jennifer completed the Nike Women's Half Marathon to benefit the Leukemia &
Lymphoma Society in 2004. She was one of the top fund-raisers in Silicon Valley.

Doctors and nurses huddled around me and told me that they
were going to perform a cardioversion to shock the heart back into
rhythm. Half out of it, I told them that there would be no cardioversion unless my cardiologist agreed. That launched a conversation with a second-year resident that was one of the most bizarre
exchanges I'd ever had:

Doctor:     Mr. Hammer, we need to shock your heart back
            into rhythm.

Me:         There will be no cardioversion.

| | |
|---|---|
| Doctor: | It is the only thing we can do for you to stop this episode. |
| Me: | Every other time this has happened, my doctors have started a drip of amiodarone or cardezim, and that seems to calm things down. |
| Doctor: | That is not what I think we should do at this time. |
| Me: | I understand that is your opinion, but not until you call my wife first and then call Dr. Al-Ahmad [my cardiologist]. |
| Doctor: | And then what; do you want us to just stand by and let you die! |

Can you imagine talking to a critically ill patient like that?

Immediately after running a half marathon, taking off her shoes, and settling into a view of the San Francisco Bay, Pamela heard her phone ringing; I told her what was happening, and she spoke with the doctor. She immediately strapped her shoes on and headed for Stanford. When Pamela returned to the hospital, she met with the attending physician on duty and made it clear that this doctor was never allowed back in my room unsupervised.

As it turned out, Dr. Al-Ahmad advised against the cardioversion and instructed that the medications be given. The episode cleared within hours—without any paddles or electric shock!

The doctor came back into the room and told his group of residents to "fold up. Our work here is done." It was clear that he was trying to show off and exert his authority. But not this day and not on this patient. Sometimes you just have to speak up for yourself and have others do so as well.

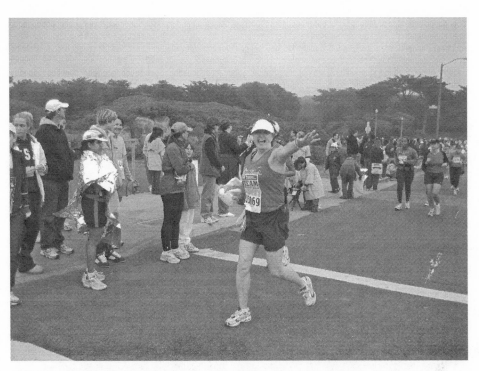

Pamela crossed the finish line at the Nike Women's Half Marathon in San Francisco in 2005 as one of northern California's top fund-raisers.

Up to this time in my life, the two most important days were the day I married Pamela and the day Gerald and Jennifer were born. I now have two more that are on an equal level: January 22, 2004 (the day of my transplant), and November 23, 2005 (the day I finally met Andrew, my donor).

Earlier in the year, I had learned that Andrew was willing to exchange his name and address with me, and we'd sent a few e-mails to each other. I learned that he had family in LA and would likely be there around Thanksgiving. Just a few short weeks before the holiday, I asked whether he and his family would be willing to come up to San Jose to see us; he enthusiastically said yes, and we sent him the tickets. He would come up the day before the holiday and spend the afternoon with us. We knew absolutely nothing about him. We had not seen any photos or heard his story, and he knew nothing about us, so that day would be full immersion from both sides.

Gerald and Jennifer were home for Thanksgiving and their birthday, and they stayed with me while Pamela drove to the airport to pick Andrew and his family up just before noon. Some of our friends would join us later, after the four of us had the opportunity to get acquainted.

Once Pamela left, I was alone with my thoughts. I did not want Gerald and Jennifer to see me, but I cried within. I did not know what to expect. I did not know what to say. How would I react? Was Andrew a macho man? If I cried would it turn him off? Was he an emotional man? What would I do if we had nothing to say to each other? Only time would tell.

When they arrived, I stood from the chair that had been my home for so many months. Just the sound of the car doors closing unleashed my emotions. After all, here was the person who had saved my life. As Andrew entered the house, we looked at each other, which lasted for seconds but seemed like an eternity. He walked over to me, but before he could take a step, I broke down. He took several steps toward me and embraced me for what was, for me, an eternity. All I could whisper (and barely audibly) was, "Thank you. I love you."

My tears flowed, seemingly forever; they just would not stop. I held in my arms a total stranger—a man who had given me life. He is much taller than me; good-looking, like me (ha ha!); and Jewish, like me. We share a similar emotional grounding, a love of family, and many other traits. Meeting him produced in me a feeling that I could not comprehend, much yet believe or explain.

We learned that our lives had crossed in only the barest of ways. Being Jewish, our ancestors were both from the Austria/Germany corner of the world, but our shared history ended there. We could not find any direct family relationship, but one never knows.

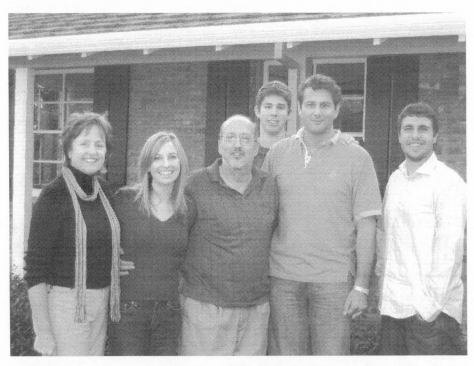

**Andrew (second from right), and his son Alexander (behind me) meet our family for the first time in San Jose.**

After getting acquainted, we learned that Andrew had registered for the bone marrow donor program ten years earlier at the suggestion of his wife, Sherry. His name sat on the registry for those years and, as he told me, he'd nearly forgotten about it. That was until one day in late 2003 when he received the phone call that would change my life forever. As Andrew describes it, he immediately agreed to be my donor and shared the good news with Sherry.

I described earlier the difficulty Andrew's donor center had had with the stem cell collection. I cannot to this day explain why he was so committed to make the donation, other than he had a sixth sense that he was truly the only lifesaver available to me; he was. There is also, in the deep recesses of my mind, the understanding that we, as Jews, have this overall moral and ethical code and commitment to our fellow men and women that transcends all and binds us together. That bond, between two people who knew nothing about each other, made happen what was a true miracle on the grandest scale between two people.

But that is not the whole story.

After we settled down to talk, I learned from Andrew that his beautiful wife, Sherry, had been diagnosed with breast cancer ten years earlier, in her early thirties. It is such a cruel disease for anyone, let alone someone so young. Together they'd fought the disease for ten years as their young son, Alexander, was growing up. As a part of her treatment, Sherry had received an autologous transplant, so they were somewhat familiar with transplants. And it was Sherry who encouraged him to be my donor and to leave her that day to travel despite the battle she was fighting.

Unfortunately, I never met Sherry; she lost her battle less than two months after Andrew saved my life. Andrew and Alexander mourn her deeply, as do Pamela, Gerald, Jennifer, and I. But we, as well as Andrew and Alexander, take some solace in knowing that before Sherry passed away, she knew that Andrew had saved someone's life. And from what I learned about her, that was the way she would have wanted it.

Words cannot express the debt of gratitude I owe to Andrew, Sherry, and Alexander. They sacrificed to give life to someone they did not know and might never meet. They gave the ultimate gift.

In my conversations with Andrew, he also made one thing clear. He will do it again if called.

What a remarkable family. They will always be my angels.

December brought yet another alarming scare. While performing a CT scan on my chest to look at the pneumonia, the doctors noticed a nodule that appeared to have the characteristics of a malignant tumor. It could be a recurrence of the leukemia or a secondary cancer. Or it could be nothing. We decided to treat it with medications (which brought some other side effects several months later) and not do a biopsy at this time. Fortunately, after two months of intense drug therapy and more tests, the nodule was determined to be a fungal infection. No cancer; just another big scare. In a cancer patient, anything unexplainable is scary.

Another bullet dodged!

Despite continuing to have issues to deal with, I was finally strong enough to have hip replacement surgery. We were referred to the head of orthopedics, Dr. William Maloney. He did a fantastic job and had me out of surgery in half of the time he had anticipated. That was important because he did not want there to be any excess bleeding or increased chance of infection.

During the surgery, Dr. Maloney discovered that I had developed avascular necrosis, which is a loss of blood flow to the hip joint. Once this begins, there is no reversing it as the bone begins to die, and the only real option is a hip replacement. Once he was inside the hip, he grabbed the ball of the joint, and it completely disintegrated in his hand. It was obvious that the replacement was long overdue; it was also clear why I was in such pain.

Most importantly, the surgery was a success, and I got out of bed four hours after returning to my room. The next morning I was walking down the hall. I was finally free of pain and able to do without the wheelchair.

I had never really understood the impact pain can have on your entire being. Since the hip break and compression fractures I had been in constant pain—for over fifteen months. It really kept me down. It further sapped my energy. It left me depressed and immobile. But once the hip was replaced and the pain abated I was a new person, almost overnight.

By the next day, I was doing a few stairs. It was almost a miracle. I felt great and prayed that I had turned a corner. Once I got home (three days earlier than expected), I was reinvigorated and renewed.

The holiday season was in full motion, and it was perhaps the most relaxed we were in a while. Although I was still ill from pneumonia and rehabilitating from the hip surgery, we were surrounded by friends. We had to continue to be careful with germs when we had small gatherings at our home (we had several). People came by regularly, and we just shared old times. Some were friends we had not seen in years. The time brought back many memories and punctuated the reason we'd decided to move back to San Jose.

As the New Year rolled in, our optimism grew. But it did not last long as I soon began to have complications, mostly related to pneumonia and lung issues. The constant pneumonias required that I receive supplemental oxygen to be able to breathe normally. Over the next several months, I went back into the hospital several times, making a total of seven hospitalizations in the first six months of 2006!

One of the hospitalizations was to fix my A-fib. Dr. Al-Ahmad performed the procedure, known as an A-fib ablation in which catheters are used to burn or ablate the electrical triggers in the heart that misfire and cause the heart beat out of rhythm and to beat rapidly. He was assisted in this procedure by a nationally reputed physician from the Cleveland Clinic who specializes in this type of problem. The procedure went extremely well, and the A-fib episodes have become few and far between.

Apparently, I could not be content on a path that did not include more hospital visits or having no major difficulties to contend with. In April 2006, I was home when I blacked out, fell, and fractured and tore a ligament in my ankle. Not only did the incident put me back in a wheelchair, it led to the diagnosis of yet another challenge: autonomic neuropathy. This is a rare condition, which probably resulted from my chemotherapy.

Autonomic neuropathy is damage to the nerves that regulate your heart rate and blood pressure, among other functions. Your nerves transmit messages between your brain and your muscles, blood vessels, skin, and internal organs. Autonomic neuropathy results in faulty communication between your brain and the parts of your body that your autonomic nervous system serves. In my case, the neuropathy resulted in not enough blood getting to my brain, which caused me to faint or black out. Now I am on medication for that, although automatic neuropathy is not curable.

As I concluded this book in late 2006, I was finishing yet another hospital stay for the outbreak of GVHD in the liver. My successor had taken over at the chamber in July, and yet another chapter in our life was turning. In August, Pamela and I celebrated our thirtieth wedding anniversary, and this was also the third anniversary of my diagnosis and, thus, of the beginning of this journey.

Complications aside, an overriding concern was simply physical conditioning. I had spent so much time in the hospital, in bed, and in a wheelchair that my physical condition was extremely low. Most of my muscles had atrophied despite physical therapy. Some of my current problems were likely the result of my conditioning status. In the months ahead, as we would begin to knock down the health issues, an improvement in conditioning will assist me dramatically in my recovery.

One vexing problem is my lungs. I developed GVHD, which manifested in a condition called bronchiolitis obliterans. Basically, many of the small airways have died off and may never recover. I am now functioning at 35 percent of normal lung capacity and on oxygen 24/7, although there is hope that this will improve, and I will only need oxygen at exertion. I pray this is so because being tethered to oxygen is no fun.

In late July of 2006, I came down unexpectedly with yet another occurrence of GVHD, this time in the liver. The result was extreme liver pain, yellow discoloration of the skin, fatigue, and related symptoms. The GVHD is under control, and Dr. Negrin placed me on a clinical trial for a new antirejection drug, but the liver problem will be with me for a long time to come; it will come and go, and we will always need to be vigilant about the symptoms. The clinical trial is for a new drug that is testing the ability to taper down the use of prednisone faster than the prior antirejection drug I was using. I have been on such high doses of prednisone for so long, and it has done so much damage to so many of my systems, that they want to test a faster taper.

I thought I would end the tracing of my journey by sharing a bit of humor I brought to the emergency room at Stanford.

During my time at Stanford, I made several trips to the emergency room for some of the issues discussed earlier. And in my own way, I also had to inject some humor into these serious occasions.

If there is one thing I have learned about going to the emergency room or the hospital—especially to a teaching hospital where interns, residents, and fellows are always learning and experimenting—is not to tell them too much. We all have aches and pains, and more often than not when I visited the hospital or emergency room, it was for something major. But I had to remember not to tell them more than they needed to know so that the residents and fellows did not try and do too much or over diagnose.

I recall one evening when Pamela and I were in the emergency room at Stanford. I had been placed on Coumadin (to thin my blood in advance of my A-fib procedure), and my blood was much too thin. I was having some unexplained bleeding, and the concern was that I could bleed to death due to the thinness of my blood. I was also having some bleeding from hemorrhoids I'd developed over the last few years but had not yet disclosed that to the doctor in the ER. When we were alone behind the curtain, Pamela said to me, "Make sure you don't tell them about your bleeding, or they will think you have colon problems and sooner than you can say 'Old McDonald Had a Farm,' you will have a three-foot long pipe going up you."

A few weeks later, we were back in the ER for similar problems. It would be yet another chance to show my sense of humor.

If you are a male over forty, you have undoubtedly had at least one DRE (digital rectal exam). They are not the most comfortable procedures, and they're slightly embarrassing.

The attending physician was a young female doctor who pronounced her intention to do the exam. Needing to relax the tension I was feeling and make things comfortable for her, I asked her to use two fingers because I wanted a second opinion! With the barest of curtains separating the beds in a busy emergency room, everyone heard the exchange and suddenly the whole room turned to riotous laughter. Sometimes humor can be the best medicine.

While some of the problems have abated, I continue to have some other issues, which will be chronic conditions that I will need to accept and deal with:

- I developed peripheral neuropathy, a second form of neuropathy, which is a condition in which I have numbness and tingling in the hands, fingers, and toes.

- I have developed GVHD in my lungs and eyes as well. The lung problem may be a lifelong problem; it's what gives me a predisposition to pneumonia and requires the oxygen. The eye GVHD causes dry eyes, and I am beginning to experience deterioration in my eyesight.

- The autonomic neuropathy is likely a permanent condition that will give me a predisposition to fainting.

- I have developed tremors that cause my hands and feet to shake.

- My energy levels continue to be low, requiring that I nap daily.

- I have severe back pain from the fractures and broken hip that limit my mobility.

- I have constant ringing in my ears that was caused by the medications I was taking for the lung lesion and will need hearing aids.

- We were forced to make a very difficult decision relating to my heart. There was only one drug that would control my A-fib. However, this drug could cause permanent lung damage in patients who had received radiation treatments. I was not strong enough to undergo the A-fib procedure until 2006, requiring that we either risk A-fib and a possible stroke or take the medicine and risk lung damage. Everyone agreed that I needed the medicine, but now it appears that I may have sustained the lung damage they were concerned about, in addition to the lung GVHD. Only time will tell whether it is a temporary or permanent condition.

- I continue to take prednisone, a very strong steroid. I need the drug to help with my lungs, but continuing to take it causes further deterioration of my bones. We don't know how we will resolve this in the long term, but it is yet another example that sometimes there are few good choices when it comes to medications.

- At last count, I have taken over two hundred fifty different medicines, received over three hundred thirty transfusions, and spent nearly six hundred nights in six different hospitals.

I decided that I would send one final farewell letter to the members of the LA political power structure, and people I had worked with as I said my good-bye to Los Angeles:

A Farewell Message from Rusty Hammer

Nearly five years ago you welcomed me with open arms as the president and CEO of the Los Angeles Area Chamber of Commerce. I arrived with high hopes knowing that this was a unique opportunity to lead the most important business organization in America's second largest city. I relished the challenge and gave it my full energy.

Unfortunately, that was interrupted when I was diagnosed with leukemia. Despite my best efforts to fight the disease and its side effects, I am no longer able to return to work full time and devote the energy required of this vital position.

I am extremely proud of what we all accomplished—the Board and its leadership, members and your professional staff. Among our many are:

- Restoring the Chamber to profitability and financial health
- Increasing membership by over 40 percent
- Merging two leadership development programs into the Chamber (Leadership L.A. and the Southern

California Leadership Network) to position us as the premiere provider of leadership training in the region

- Developing a strategic partnership with UNITE-LA to position us squarely at the leading edge of education reform

- Being the voice for business through our enormously successful and award-winning Business Perspective

- Expanding the Access Sacramento trip to 100 participants and Access D.C. to 70 (from 12 when we first started)

- Developing new, compelling, and award-winning publications

- Continuing to set attendance records at all of our events

- Creating the Civic Medal of Honor to shine a light on individuals who have distinguished themselves with a lifetime of service to our region

- Bringing World Trade Week under the auspices of the Chamber

- Creating Mobility 21, a coalition of business, labor, government and community groups to advocate for our transportation needs

- Creating the highly successful Pancakes and Politics

- Restoring the pride and honor of the Chamber

There is much more to do—and much more that will be done as we pursue our Strategic Plan. I know that the board, management, and staff are poised to keep the momentum going forward.

I am disappointed that I will not be able to lead the organization through the planning we have completed and the growth we anticipate. There are still things left undone that I wanted to accomplish. I will continue to be involved with the Chamber as a Senior Policy Advisor, counseling on public policy and political issues of the day.

Unfortunately, this disease and its never-ending complications have gotten the best of me—for now. Although I will continue helping the Chamber as a Senior Policy Advisor, my career as your president and CEO will come to an end on June 30.

My successor is Gary Toebben, from Northern Kentucky. He is a career chamber professional, and a good friend who will serve you well.

I close by extending my thanks for the time we had together. It was a pleasure—indeed, an honor—to have been chosen for this important position. I will miss it dearly and I will miss L.A. What I will miss most is all of you. The love, compassion, and well wishes you extended to me and my family during the darkest days were appreciated more than you will ever know.

I wish to extend special thanks to those who have served as my colleagues and mentors, both officers and staff who filled in when I was not able to do so.

I extend to the Chamber, its leadership, Board, members and staff my very best wishes for the future. I hope that a time will come when we are able to work together, and I hope you will please stay in touch.

Thank you, and best wishes,

Russell J. "Rusty" Hammer
President & CEO

It is my firm hope that I have had all the major surgeries and procedures I will need and that my future will focus on healing and recovery—and on my new life.

Despite the pain and complications, I remain positive about my experience because I am alive and able to pursue my goals and be here for my family, friends, and loved ones.

It has been nearly three years since we first heard the C word. It has been a long road of uncertainty, hospitalizations, needles, tests, medications, and near-death experiences. I pray that the worst is over, and somehow I feel as though it is. But I also know that the future is unpredictable. I do not know from one day to the next how I will feel. I fight and struggle and I intend to maintain the optimism that things will get better in the months and years ahead and that I will attain the recovery that we have dreamed about.

> This time, like all times, is a very good one
> if we but know what to do with it.
> —Ralph Waldo Emerson[23]

As the month came to an end, Pamela decided that we would attempt what would be our first extended outing in three years; we would spend several days at the beach courtesy of Sal and Barbara's mother. They have a home at Pajaro Dunes (the site of our honeymoon).

Although I was not able to go into the water (too many stairs down to the beach), I made it to the sand once and out on the patio. What struck me more than anything was reflecting back on the past thirty years. As I said at the beginning, when we were first there Pamela and I were transfixed by the birds gliding over the water, the beautiful sunsets, and the unending horizon that seemed to open the world and its endless opportunities to us.

The birds are still there. The air is still fresh. The sunsets are as beautiful and the horizon still beckons its limitless call to us. While our burdens are greater and our cares about the future different, the endless call of the seas, the ocean and its unending boundary still calls out to us; it gives us life; it gives us hope.

That is what we will cling to as we write the next chapter of our life.

23   http://www.quotationspage.com/quote/39018.html

# PART II

# IMPROVING THE JOURNEY

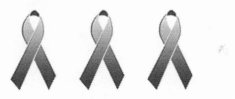

# CHAPTER 4

# IF YOU ARE DIAGNOSED WITH CANCER

*Live Like You Are Dying*[24]

And a moment came that stopped me on a dime …
I hope you get the chance to live like you were dying.
—Tim McGraw

As the adage goes, on your deathbed you probably will not wish that you had spent more time at the office.

Like the man in Tim McGraw's song, I received news one day that stopped me on a dime. It was news that told me that I was dying. Unfortunately, it happens to too many people every day all around the world. The lives of too many people and their families are torn apart every day by unexpected diagnoses of cancer and other life-threatening illnesses. Such a diagnosis is hard to deal with. Sometimes it is too late. But many times it is in time. Hopefully,

---

24  http://www.lyrics007.com/Tim%20McGraw%20Lyrics/Live%20Like%20You%20
Were%20Dying%20Lyrics.html

some of the things I have laid out in this book will help people to be more prepared to deal with the uncertainties and realities of dealing with these matters. Some people actually get the chance to live like they were dying rather than regret not having done so.

The day you learn you have cancer will change your life forever. Immediate thoughts of death will overcome you.

You may blame yourself for your cancer, especially if you have risk factors that you could have prevented, such as having been a smoker. You will worry about your family. You will imagine harsh treatments and pain. You will step from a world of familiarity to one of uncertainty. Everything that influences your daily life—from your job and finances to your family, relationships, and friends—will change overnight. You will lose control over most parts of your life as you surrender to doctors, clinics, hospitals, and all of the other aspects of fighting your disease. But if all these changes cause you to give up and think that your life is already over, you will be making a big mistake. Even if your life ends up being limited, there are still many things that you can do in the time you have.

Cancer can do many things to your mental state, and you will need to remain focused. It will steal many things from you, but if you focus positively you will find that:

- Cancer will not steal your family

  They will always be by your side in ways that you cannot predict or understand.

- Cancer will not destroy your hope

  Hope comes from within yourself and from what others transmit to you. It is within your control.

- <u>Cancer will not take away your courage</u>

  You alone have the power to mount the courage you will need for this battle.

- <u>Cancer will not suppress memories of good times</u>

  In fact, holding on to the memory of good times and resolving to relive them—and to make more memories—will keep you going.

- <u>Cancer will not destroy your mind</u>

  In all but the rarest cases of cancers that affect the brain, you will find that you are as strong intellectually as you have always been. In fact, you may find even greater capacities for knowledge as you compensate for any physical limitations.

- <u>Cancer alone will not kill your spirit</u>

  Stay positive. Don't let it get the best of you.

- <u>Cancer will not destroy your faith</u>

  Keep your faith—in whatever way you express faith.

Cancer clearly is an injustice. It is not fair. It attacks good people. But a fact of life is that the vast majority of us will get it or will know people who do. Cancer separates those who have had it from those who have not in ways you cannot imagine. Despite people's attempts to "understand what you are going through" and to "sympathize with your situation," nobody can truly understand who has not dealt with it themselves—not even those who have had a serious illness.

Cancer may well strike in the prime of your life, often unexpectedly, and there are few things you could have done about it. As one transplant survivor said:

> I think the emotional effects of getting diagnosed
> with cancer are deep.
> It's like a wound that never heals.[25]

In the beginning, it is important to remember that cancer is not the end of the world—nor is it the end of your life. But it is the beginning of a new world for you—and the beginning of a different life. Your world and your life will never be the same again. Do not focus on the fact that things will never be the same, focus instead in the fact that things will be different, and resolve that you will make something positive of your new and different life.

You must believe that your cancer is potentially a growing experience because it will make you a better person. It will teach you more about yourself, your values, and courage than almost any other experience you will have in your life. And I guarantee you that it will bring you closer to friends and family, will help you to become more sensitive and more in touch with the things that are important in your life and in the lives of others.

You need to have faith in the future. Things may not work out as you planned, but cancer will give you a new chance to plan. Your earnings may be different. Your career challenges may be different. You may live differently. But facing such fundamental turns

---

25  Fred Hutchinson Cancer Research Center. Long Term Follow Up Program, *Thoughts and Comments from Patients*

in the road of life can also be a refreshing chance to embrace new opportunities.

The care of someone with a life-threatening illness is, as I have suggested, not something that can be engaged in only by doctors, or by health care professionals alone for that matter. It must involve all elements of a patient's world—most critically the patient himself or herself and the patient's caregiver or advocate who can interpret and communicate for the patient. I know from firsthand experience that, as a patient, I was often so exhausted and forlorn that I could not ask the right questions, much less engage in a discussion about my treatment, or argue when things were not going right.

I saw too many examples of patients going along to get along. We heard too many stories about families who sat quietly by and trusted the treatments to doctors. And, while patients must do so ultimately, there are a number of things they can do as well to improve patient care:

- Have a positive mental attitude.

  This is one of the most powerful tools in your arsenal against cancer that is totally within your control. As Patricia Neal said, "A strong positive mental attitude will create more miracles than any wonder drug."[26] Your mind is powerful and can overcome many things, including physical pain and despair, so use your mind to overcome obstacles.

---

26  http://www.quoteworld.org/quotes/9333

- <u>Be at your best before treatment begins.</u>

  The better shape and condition you are in at the beginning of treatment, the better shape you will be when it is over. Remember, no matter what treatment you have, you will lose weight. You won't be as active, so it is better to be in good shape before you begin.

- <u>Take some time off or go on a vacation.</u>

  If you have the option, get away, even for a short time. You will be able to relax and spend some quality time with your family before the onslaught begins. You will begin your treatment with good memories and in a good frame of mind. You will also make good new memories that you can call upon during your treatment. We went to Europe as a family and had a wonderful time, even though clouds gathered over our heads. As I look back on things, it was one of the best things we did for ourselves.

- <u>Read inspirational materials and listen to uplifting tapes/music.</u>

  Read about good experiences from cancer patients and talk to some survivors. This will give you confidence that the battle can be won.

- <u>Don't dwell in anger or ask, why me?</u>

  The fact of the matter is that it is you and you must deal with your cancer. All energy you spend on the anger and the negative saps your ability to focus that same energy on the positive things in your life—your family, etc.—and on the process of healing and recovery. You must remember that, no matter what people may do for you to be of help, you are the most important part of your own healing—as important as or more important than your doctors because it will take every ounce of your will to heal in addition to all of their medicines and expertise.

Most importantly, you must remember that you are entering a *new* phase of your life, not the last phase. An important part of living in this new phase is to put you first. You may be a person who has always done things for others, taken care of others, and provided for your family. These dynamics may well change. You must begin to take care of yourself. You must assume responsibility for your own wellness, for you are the most important person who can make a difference in your own health. But you must also cross an important line—you must be willing to accept the fact that other people will now be taking care of you just as you have taken care of them.

Hopefully, you will have a caregiver who will do many things that you will not be able to do for yourself. You may need to turn over tasks at work to others. You may not be able to work. Your income may change. Your lifestyle may change. But this is not the end. You may be fortunate enough to go through your cancer journey and complete it with little change; if so you will be extremely fortunate. But, if not, always remember that your cancer will be a bridge to a new phase in your life, not the end of it.

- <u>Identify a caregiver.</u>

  As early as possible, identify someone in your close circle of friends or family who can serve as your caregiver.
  This should be a person who can accompany you to all
  (or most) doctor appointments, tests, or treatments. You
  will find that your recollection of tests, treatments, medications, progress reports, etc. will be sketchy because you
  simply cannot focus on everything that is said to you. The
  old adage, two heads are better than one, is true. You will
  also find that you will be tired and simply won't be able to
  keep up. The person you identify will have the important
  responsibility of being your eyes and ears, keeping a journal, and making sure that you understand what is happening with your treatment. In this regard, try and centralize
  all notes in one notebook. Have an index that allows you
  to keep good records.

  This is an awesome commitment that someone will make
  to you, but it is absolutely essential that you find someone
  who can do so. Think of this person as the commanding
  general for your battle. This person will call many of the
  shots, set the strategy, and assure that the army does its
  job. This person will need to put a portion of their life on
  hold and help you through your difficult journey. In my
  case, my caregiver was my wife, Pamela, and I can tell you
  that I would not be alive today without her.

- Keep a medication journal.

  Make certain that your journal has a separate section that contains information about all medications you have taken, the dosages, frequencies, and specifically any reactions you have had to these medications. This information will prove invaluable to you and your medical team months and years down the road.

- Learn everything you can about your disease.

  Know the language of your disease. You will find, in most areas of endeavor and perhaps in medicine more than in any other, there is a whole new language. Learn it. Know the acronyms. Ask for and consume as much information as you can. Know something about the tests you will be undergoing. Know your medications: know what they are used for and know what they look like. If you don't understand what someone is trying to say, don't pretend as if you do; ask them to talk to you in layman's language. All of these things will make it easier to understand your disease, your treatment, and what to expect along the way. You may wish to refer to the web site I have developed that provides links to what I think are helpful Internet sites, at www.CancerWebLinks.com

  The Internet is an excellent resource for obtaining information about your diagnosis and treatment options, but it can be a bottomless pit of information. Look for major organizational Web sites, such as the organization that specializes in your disease (the Leukemia & Lymphoma

Society, the American Lung Association, etc.). Contact the disease-specific organizations that deal with your illness to determine how they can help you.

You should also consider printing information from reliable Internet sites about your disease and keeping the information with your journal. Ask your doctor for these materials as well.

- Identify an advocate.

  This could be a duty of your caregiver or of a second person. Either way, the role of an advocate is equally vital. Your advocate needs to be there to speak for you when you can't. There will be times when your advocate needs to ask tough questions of your doctors and nurses. Decisions will need to be reviewed, questioned, and challenged. If you are hospitalized, an advocate is critical in order to make sure you receive the priority and quality of care you deserve.

- Obtain other opinions.

  Even the finest medical centers, doctors, and labs can make errors. Doctors can have different opinions. New therapies are developed every day that not every doctor may know about. It would be irresponsible to begin a course of treatment without getting additional opinions—both on the diagnosis as well as on the treatment options. In the end, you will decide the course of your treatment, and you should only do so after becoming as informed as you can be.

- <u>Take control of your treatment.</u>

  You will find that there are many options, and you alone will be the one enduring the outcomes. Don't go down a road unless you are prepared for the consequences. In addition, make sure that every test, whether invasive or not, is absolutely essential. You should not undergo tests unless they are necessary and the test will give you information needed by your doctors that can only be gained through the tests being ordered.

- <u>Ask questions until you have no more.</u>

  Remember, it is your body. It is your life. Therefore, anything that is done is done for and to you. So you must be in control of the treatment that is being done. Do not let the doctors or the medical team do anything that you do not want them to do. Ask questions about everything, and, if you are not satisfied with the answers, do not authorize procedures to be done or tests to be taken.

- <u>Pay attention to your lab results.</u>

  Get to know what the major lab results mean and how your numbers are tracking. You can often spot changes that others may not see.

- <u>Select the best doctors you can identify.</u>

  Consult your local medical association. Look at your potential doctors' résumés. Make sure that they have specific expertise in (and preferably that they have conducted research and written papers on) your disease.

- <u>Know your medicines.</u>

  As a patient, you have a responsibility to know something about the medicine you are taking. What is the name of the medicine? What is its purpose? What does it look like? What are its possible side effects? Does it interact with anything else you are taking? How often do you take it? What do you do if you miss a dose?

  You should develop a medication chart that lists all medicines, dosages, and the frequency you take them. I suggest that you check off each drug when you take it so that you do not miss anything. Many drugs must be taken consistently at the same time each day, and a chart will ensure that you do not stray from the prescription.

  Furthermore, you should always carry with you a list of each medicine you are taking, including its strength and the frequency with which you are taking it. Every time you go to any doctor, he or she will review your medications, and carrying a list will be especially helpful in the case of an unanticipated hospitalization as the hospital will want a complete listing.

  I have too many stories of drug errors that have been made in the hospital, specifically with me. It does no good to blame a nurse for giving you the wrong medicine or not giving you something you are supposed to take. Nurses have many patients and lots of medicine to give—although they are careful, they can sometimes make mistakes. Remember, it is your mouth that swallows the pills and your body that reacts to them, and you must take on the responsibility of knowing which medications you should be taking and when as well. Two heads are better than one!

Beyond this, it is important that you understand the risks of medications. You will be taking so many, which will often be prescribed by different physicians, that it could be easy to wind up taking medications that are contraindicated. That is why it is essential that each of your doctors must know all of the medications you are taking.

Reading the information sheets on drugs can be confusing and technical. In addition, they contain cautions about things that happen in a very small percentage of patients taking the drugs. But it never hurts to understand the potential for problems.

You must also understand that sometimes there are no good answers when it comes to medications. I have several examples of this. Transplant patients take prednisone, a strong steroid. But prednisone causes lots of side effects and complications. It is probably why I developed osteoporosis and diabetes. But I needed the prednisone to survive.

I was taking a strong antibiotic called vancomycin. It was essential, but we knew that it might (and did) cause hearing damage. But I needed the drug.

Finally, I needed to take medication to control my A-fib, and the only thing that worked was amiodarone. However, that drug can be toxic to the lungs of patients who have received radiation. But we had no choice, and now I am fighting a battle against poor lung function. These were cases in which there were no good choices, but a choice was necessary nonetheless.

- <u>Select the best facility</u>.

  If you will avail yourself of a medical center or a NCI designated Comprehensive Cancer Center, make sure the facility has specific expertise in your particular disease. For example, I recall the tragic case of someone who became a friend of mine; we will call him Jack. I met Jack only on the phone through a friend. He had leukemia and had undergone an autologous transplant, which unfortunately had not worked. He was then facing the need for an allogeneic transplant and, fortunately, a donor was identified. The medical center that performed his autologous transplant had a good history with those transplants but had only recently begun allogeneic transplants. I urged him as forcefully as I could to switch to another facility that has extensive allogeneic transplant experience; however, he chose to remain where he was. Allogeneic transplants are very different in their protocols, medications, and as importantly in the side effects that patients will incur specifically GVHD complications (and necessarily the treatment of these complications).

Unfortunately for Jack, he developed complications after the allogeneic transplant, and the outcome was tragic. I can't say that he would have lived if he was at a different facility, but I know that he probably would have increased his chances had he been at a facility with much more extensive experience with the type of transplant he needed.

- Understand your insurance coverage.

  Before you get too far, make sure you understand your insurance coverage. This includes health insurance, disability insurance, and any other type of insurance you may have. Make sure your health insurance company assigns you a case manager to work with you to maximize your benefits. Your hospital or cancer facility should do the same to make sure that the insurance company is billed for and pays for all of its obligations.

- Set up a way to communicate.

  If you can, ask a friend or family member to set up an e-mail list to your friends, family, and associates to keep them informed of your progress. Karen did this for me, and it was one of the best things that could have been done. We were instantly able to communicate the ups and downs, and more importantly it became easy for people to get messages of support and hope to me just when I needed them. You will never really know how many people your life has touched until you have cancer. You will be amazed at the number of people who come to your aid and who want to be of help. Remember, it is not the big things that people can do for you; it is the little things. Receiving a call or a note card or e-mail or just knowing someone cares is enough to give you the strength to persevere.

- <u>Keep your own diary or journal.</u>

  One important lesson I learned is the importance of keeping a diary or journal. I have reconstructed my experiences as best as I could, but I did not have the benefit of a daily journal. That is partially because I had a rough treatment course and, for days or weeks at a time, had no ability to record my experiences. Chemotherapy, in my opinion, is the roughest treatment that medicine can impose on an individual. It literally and figuratively takes a person to the door of death and (hopefully) brings him or her back. The patient is often semiconscious or out of it for days at a tine. Constipation, diarrhea, fevers, sweats, and chills interrupt any moments of good feelings. Keeping a diary under these circumstances can be difficult.

  I have found that there are lapses in my memory—things about which I have little recognition—so I urge you to try your best to make your own record anyhow. Show the discipline I did not have and keep a diary or journal (or ask someone to do it for you).

Write down everything from appointment notes and contact information for doctors and hospitals to test dates and test results, to what you ate for dinner and how your caregiver's smile warmed you up after a long night. Every detail is important. It will be helpful in remembering your journey and could be of great assistance to your doctors in cataloging side effects and correlating them with changes in medications or other treatments. It is critical to record how you are feeling, at least on a daily basis. This will help correlate problems you are having with medications you took, treatments you underwent, foods you ate, etc. If, for example, you see a doctor every few weeks and tell them, "Last Tuesday I had a problem with …," having a journal that records what you were doing at the time and what you did about it will help your doctor solve the puzzle. Absent that, you and your physician will be guessing.

- <u>Know your symptoms.</u>

  Be conscious of your body. Know whether that pain in your neck is just a muscle pain from sleeping wrong or whether it is more serious. I recall one episode where I had intense pain in my neck and wrote it off as sore muscles from physical therapy that I had just started the day earlier. But the pain was intense, and Pamela felt that something was wrong. She pressed the doctors to investigate further, and they discovered that I had a life-threatening staph infection that had settled around the catheter in my neck.

- <u>Celebrate the small stuff.</u>

  You will find days during your treatment and recovery when there are big victories. A negative PET scan or biopsy are examples of big things to celebrate. But on most days, your victories will be much smaller—walking a block, just getting out of bed, preparing a meal. Those things may seem small, but remember, you are running a marathon, not a sprint. So if you celebrate a collection of small victories, you will soon find yourself down the marathon track.

- <u>Manage your pain.</u>

  You will find that cancer is a painful disease. You may experience pain from the tumor locations. You will probably get headaches, joint pain, bone aches, and other pain from medications. If you are in bed for an extensive period of time, you may get back pain. Don't be like me. I was the macho type; I kept saying that I didn't need pain medications, until it was too late. I used to say, "I'll be fine," or "Don't worry, I am OK," or other expressions that minimized my needs. Everything that you do for yourself and everything that you expend energy on that other people can do for you takes away energy you can use to rest, heal, and recover. I learned that unless you get ahead of the pain curve, it will overtake you, and it is difficult to get back on top. There is nothing wrong with asking for pain medications. It does not make you look weak!

- Get lots of rest.

   Unless you are at your best, your body will not fight as hard as it can. The key to being the best you can be given your limitations is having the rest and energy you need every day to fight your battle.

- Demand the best from everyone.

   You deserve nothing less than the best doctors, the best hospitals, the best technicians, and the best nurses. If you don't get the best, say so. If you see an unsafe practice, report it. If your blood is being drawn, and a technician fails to wash his or her hands and/or wear gloves, stop him or her. If someone is discourteous or unresponsive, let someone know. You are in the fight for your life; you deserve nothing less than the best people have to offer.

- Don't try to be tough.

   Don't try to impress anyone. Everyone understands that you are in a tough battle and that you can only do what you can do. Don't stretch yourself too far or waste your energy on anything other than recovery.

- Ask questions until you have no more.

   Remember, your interactions with your doctors will be among the most important discussions you will ever have. Approach them like you would a business meeting or other important event. Prepare! Write down questions in advance. Know what you want to get from the discussions. Don't go in half prepared, or you will come away with less information than you should. Here are some questions you should ask early on.

- What kind of cancer do I have?

- Has it spread to other areas, or is it confined?

- Do I need additional tests? If so, which ones do you recommend?

- Who would you suggest I consult for a second opinion?

- What treatment choices do I have?

- When should I begin my treatment?

- What are the consequences if I postpone treatment?

- How many patients do you see each year with cases like mine?

- If I was your relative, what would you recommend I do?

- What side effects are there to the treatments that you recommend?

- What can I do to help reduce the side effects I may have?

- How much pain will I have, and how will you treat it?

- When will I be able to go back to work?

- What drugs will I be receiving, and what are the possible side and aftereffects?

- What are the chances that my cancer will come back once I am in remission?

- What is the outlook for my survival?

- What is your view of the role of social workers and support as a part of my total treatment?

- What will be my quality of life after treatment?

- Are you board certified and licensed?

- Are you a member of any professional societies?

- (For those of you who are facing a leukemia or blood cancer diagnosis) Is your hospital or cancer center experienced in blood cancers? Will I need a stem cell transplant? Are there hospitals in our area that do the type of transplant I will need? Are there any other oncologists specializing in blood-related cancers with whom you would recommend I speak?

- Are you or a member of your staff always available in case I have questions or problems?

- Will there be nurses, social workers, and case managers available to help me with my physical needs and qual-ity-of-life concerns?

- Am I eligible for a clinical trial? Are there any clinical trials available through your hospital, center, or clinic?

- <u>Think ahead before weekends and holidays.</u>

  One thing we learned somewhat the hard way, although it may sound tongue in cheek, is that you should avoid getting sick on weekends and holidays. But it is true. The regular medical staff, especially your doctor, is likely not on service on those days, and you usually are dealing with relief staff who do not know you or your case. Therefore, as weekends and holidays approach, make sure you ask who will be on duty and make sure that proper instructions are left so the staff is adequately briefed

- <u>Talk to other patients.</u>

  Try to find someone who has been through your "specific" disease. For example, although I had leukemia, the treatments and side effects for AML are different than for other leukemias. So it was important to find people who had been through AML with chemo, radiation, and an unrelated transplant.

  That having been said, remember that your experience will not be like anyone else's. So, by talking to other patients, you will get a feel for what to expect, but your experience will be different.

- <u>Join a support group.</u>

  Talk with other patients about what you are going through. These groups can be of tremendous value in helping you cope with your disease by allowing you to talk through your problems and challenges and realize that other people are going through the same challenges. You will also stumble upon pieces of advice that will help you. And go as often as you can.

- Take things one day at a time.

  You can't do anything about yesterday and don't know what will happen tomorrow, so it is best to face the issues facing you and adapt to your condition on a daily basis blocking out the past bad memories and resolving to make today the best day.

- Be honest with others.

  If your prognosis is uncertain, tell your family, loved ones, and friends. But if you know that your time is limited, make sure they know that as well. Nothing would be worse than to set up an expectation that is false, for that would deprive you and your loved ones of obtaining closure—of saying and doing those things you would have done if they had known.

  This is especially true when dealing with children. Although I am no social worker, in my experience, I have seen that depending on their age, young ones have an ability to understand and adapt in ways we cannot imagine. Two examples help in this regard.

  My mother was with us in Florida and was very ill. We knew that she did not have long to live. Gerald and Jennifer were thirteen at the time, and we sent them to a planned week-long camp. My mother died when they were away, but we decided not to send for them; instead we waited until they returned to tell them. We only recently learned that they were very angry that they were not called to be home with their grandma the day she died. They wanted to be there.

Earlier I wrote that Pamela's brother, Jerry, died from leukemia as a young boy. Pamela remembers that her parents told her brother and her that Jerry was sick and that he had gone into the hospital a few times, but they were never told he was dying. She saw him one evening in the hospital, and the next morning a neighbor woke her and her brother up to tell them that Jerry had passed away. She says that she will never get over not knowing that he was going to die and not having said good-bye.

- Never give up.

    People around you won't, and if they see you give up, they will lose hope. Never lose faith that you will improve—no matter what faith you hold dear. Holding on to your faith and keeping hope alive will provide you with the energy you will need to get through each day.

    One transplant survivor wrote, "Long-term leukemia-free survival, that's the goal. I'm at the year-and-six months post transplant. If I make it five years, I've got a pretty good shot of living longer."[27]

---

27  Fred Hutchinson Cancer Research Center. Long Term Follow Up Program, *Thoughts and Comments from Patients*

Know that your friends and family are there to support you, and reach out to them. I had a hard time because all of my life I had taken care of others and watched out for my family, and it was foreign for me to expect others to do that for me. But I learned that they wanted to, and I realized that I would do it for them. Just as you should not take life for granted, you should never take the people in your life for granted. They will do anything for you. I often said that I was not really concerned about me because I knew the hospital would look after me. I was concerned about who would take care of my friends and family. Who would make sure they were safe? Who would hold their hands? Who would keep them sane? How would they do what they need to do every day and still be there for me?

What I learned is that friends and family lay themselves down for you. They care less about themselves during these crises. They rise to the level of angels.

- Don't put things off.

  True, the adage, don't put off until tomorrow what you can do today is cliché, and all of us have probably said it at one time or another. But its importance becomes clear once you are diagnosed with a terminal illness. I never appreciated it until I was told that my life might come to an end sooner than I'd expected. We all have a duty to ourselves and our families to make the most out of life that we can, and putting off things until tomorrow or not making the best out of your life that you can is cheating yourself and your family, friends, and community. I urge you to never put off until tomorrow what you can do today. I encourage you to never assume that you will get to something important next week—because there may never be a next week. I beg you to never end a day angry with a loved one.

- Don't cheat yourself.

  You are the most important aspect of your own recovery, and you must keep that at the forefront of your thoughts. This was perhaps the most challenging thing I had to deal with. My tendency to do too much for others often resulted in cheating myself of needed time to heal. This is a cycle that you do not want to get your self trapped into.

- Don't rush back to work too soon.

  Don't do more than you can do. Take advantage of people who want to do things for you. Spend all of the time you need focusing on building your emotional and physical strength. Getting back to anything that resembles normal may take longer than you want, but I assure you that you will be stronger and more ready to cope if you wait to return to the routine until you're absolutely ready. Going back to work too soon will set you back in ways you cannot imagine.

- Be open with doctors; tell them everything.

  You must be honest with your doctors. If you have questions, ask them. If you want a second opinion from another doctor, your physician will not be insulted if he or she is confident in him or herself. If you want to go in a different direction than your physician recommends, do not be afraid to say so.

Although I disagree somewhat with the survivor I quote below, I believe that communicating too much at one time will give your physicians too much to work on. So I suggest that you focus on what is bothering you the most and, as things play out, talk about lesser issues as well. I don't believe in hiding things from your doctors, but I don't think you should complain about everything lest you be seen as crying wolf.

In one transplant survivor's words, "Never keep anything from your doctor. If you're experiencing pain, discomfort, a strange symptom, don't assume it's supposed to be that way. Tell your doctor. If you keep something from them it could hurt your treatment, and might end up coming back to haunt you. If you feel discomfort, tell them. If you feel pain, tell them. It may be something that's not supposed to happen, or it may not be anything at all."[28]

- Communicate.

    Don't be afraid to tell people how you feel. You need to temper that with reporting both the positive and the negative. If you always talk about the negative and the pain and the mental issues you are confronting, people will get tired and discouraged. So mix some good news in with the bad. Even the smallest things (like having gotten out of bed or

---

28  Fred Hutchinson Cancer Research Center. Long Term Follow Up Program, *Thoughts and Comments from Patients*

waking up without a headache or not being in pain) give hope to others.

- <u>Don't fear the mumbo jumbo.</u>

  Sometimes I feel as though the medical community needs to follow a simple practice: perform helpful random acts of speaking English (PHRASE). You will find out, if you don't know it already, that doctors speak in a highly technical language. Many do it as a defense mechanism—to show you that they know more than you. But don't let them do that. Ask them to speak in plain English so that you understand what they are saying.

  For your assistance I have included a cancer glossary in the appendices. This glossary contains some of the many terms you will hear along with definitions. These are not medical-dictionary-quality definitions, but the glossary will help you gain an initial understanding of the many terms that you will hear.

- <u>Keep up a sense of humor.</u>

  I guarantee it will get you through the toughest days and deepest valleys. I overcame some of my toughest days and roughest conversations by expressing my sense of humor. It is a great healer, and a great way to relieve tension.

  "What has helped me the most to get past the difficulties of transplant and subsequent illnesses is to surround myself with positive minded people and have a sense of humor. I

choose to look on the bright side and be grateful for whatever time I may have left and not dwell on the negative,"[29]
noted one transplant recipient.

- <u>Take care of yourself.</u>

  I cannot emphasize enough that you are the most important element in your survival and recovery. All of the drugs
  and treatments that medicine has to offer will be inadequate in the face of a patient who does not display the will
  and mental strength to survive.

- <u>Support your caregiver.</u>

  The job of a caregiver is tough. Note that I called it a job.
  Pamela and I have learned that you can't do it part time; it
  becomes a fulltime commitment. When I say full time, I don't
  mean eight hours a day; I mean twenty-four hours a day,
  seven days a week. Caregivers are always thinking about the
  patient. When they are home alone at night and the patient
  is in the hospital, they never know when the phone will ring.
  When the patient is home, caregivers can't help but be awakened at all hours each time his or her patient turns in bed,
  gets up, or has problems that need to be attended to.


  But caregivers need to be at their best both physically and
  emotionally in order to be of most value to the patient.
  Therefore, it is important for a caregiver to find a support group to share stories, issues, and tears. And caregivers must take care of themselves physically as well. Pamela

---

29   Ibid.

made exercise a daily priority in order to have the physical and mental release she needed during this difficult time.

- Ignore unfavorable statistics.

  You are your own unique individual with your own set of challenges and treatments—not a statistic on a piece of paper. I have quoted some statistics in this book but am mindful of what Mark Twain and Benjamin Disraeli once said: "There are three types of lies: lies, dam lies, and statistics."[30]

  That is not to say that statistics are not important; it only says that statistics can be manipulated. Statistics are important in giving an indication of trends, but I urge you to not dwell on them. Dwelling on statistics can be depressing, and that is not something a patient should entertain. And, as a part of having the positive mental attitude you need to get through your ordeal, resolve that you will not be a statistic. Resolve that your case is special and that you will beat the stats.

- Take charge.

  Remember, you are in charge of your own healing and wellness. So take charge. Don't leave it for others. Nobody is more interested in your wellness than you are.

- Be assertive and trust your instincts.

  You must be assertive as a patient, and your caregiver must be assertive as well. If you are not comfortable with a given test that is planned, say so. If you are concerned about tak-

---

30   http://en.wikipedia.org/wiki/Lie "Etiquette of Lying"

ing a medication, make sure your doctor knows. If you want something, ask for it. Don't sit back and do something that, in your gut or your heart, troubles you. It may be that you need it, but make sure you talk it out first.

- Make sure your papers are in order.

  In addition to having your medication sheets with you, there are two other documents you should always carry—and always have in the hospital. The first is an advanced directive that complies with your state law that describes your final wishes. I know that the necessity of writing an advanced directive is difficult for some people to think about, but preparing one is necessary and could save your loved ones from having to make very hard decisions on which they may not agree. Advanced directives spell out how far you want to go with treatments as they pertain to sustaining life, and most hospitals now ask you for one now upon admission. Put someone in charge of making decisions for you should you become unable to make your own decisions, and make sure that person knows what you want. That person should follow the advanced directives document, which spells out how far you want to go with treatments and what lengths you want medical providers to go to as well as directing what should happen in the event that things don't go well—what your final wishes are. It is easier to have these discussions and make these decisions when not facing them in real time.

Doing so is painful—absolutely. But if you have advanced directives, it could relieve your loved ones of the pain of guessing what you would want to do.

Secondly, you should have a power of attorney that grants legal authority on your behalf. Because of various laws to protect patient confidentiality, the flow of information about your condition or status as a patient in the absence of a power of attorney or legal authorization is quite limited. So make sure that you have your legal documents in order to assure your proper care and provide for your wishes.

You should also keep with you the names and phone numbers of key family members, your caregiver, and other members of your team.

- Question everyone.

  I used to be a medicine man: I believed that medicine can cure it all. I believed that you should take the word of your doctor. I didn't question anything. I still believe that doctors are the most critical part of the team—their knowledge, education, and experience are paramount. But because of my experience, I now know that medicine can only go so far. The best medicines, procedures, surgeries, and treatments in the world cannot save you if you do not want to be saved. And that means that patients must take their own wellness into their own hands.

You, as a patient must summon all that is within you, especially in the case of cancer, to want to survive. You are engaged in a battle for your life and will need all of the courage, will power, and determination to get through what will be some of the harshest days of your life. Essential elements of this portion of the battle include summoning the support of friends who will encourage you and having faith that you will survive (and I don't mean just religious faith; I mean whatever gives you faith, hope, and confidence). These will get you through.

At the same time, and not to bring you down, it is also important to be realistic. You must pray (or whatever you do) for the best but plan for the worst. Have conversations with loved ones about what will happen if things don't go well. Plans for services and final wishes should not be thought of as morbid; you need to think of them as loving ways of helping your family, relieving them of a great burden, and doing for you what you would want done for yourself.

# CHAPTER 5

# IF YOU ARE THE FRIEND OF A CANCER PATIENT

*You've Got a Friend*[31]

You just call out my name, and you know wherever I am,
I'll come running ...
—James Taylor

James Taylor sang those words about the importance of friendships. The lyrics express how my friends reacted to my illness and how I hope yours will if ever you find yourself in trouble. I have learned more from my friends about commitment and dedication—and friendship—than I have ever taught them.

I was so fortunate that I was able to call upon so many friends who came to our assistance during this time. I didn't really call upon them as much as they came to us, and that is a big distinction. Many of them were people who came out of the woodwork from days long past; many were those we regularly associated with.

---

31  http://www.lyricsfreak.com/j/james+taylor/youve+got+a+friend_20069226.html

They have given of themselves unselfishly in so many ways, and in ways that we never expected. They really made a difference, and if you maintain your friendships, you will find that those relationships will pay off in huge rewards in your life as well.

It was very difficult to talk with my family about my disease, and it was just as tough to inform our many friends. From those I have known since elementary school to those we met along our travels through life, many people have become great supporters and lifelong friends. My friends played a huge role in keeping me optimistic and encouraging me to fight on.

It is difficult to single out people from so many friends that came to our side. Earlier I mentioned that I received over a thousand cards, e-mails, and calls. I cannot talk about each of them, and doing so would be tedious for you as well. In an appendix, I have listed all of those people who wrote or called. Peruse the list and you may see some names you will recognize. I certainly wanted to honor all of them by recognizing them in the book. But some of them I recognize below to give you an idea of some of the things you can do for someone who is ill.

I wrote a lot about the friendship we share with Steve, Karen, and Sam. They were tremendously supportive of our family and of me.

I remember one day when my friend from elementary school, Mark, gave me a baseball autographed by Willie Mays to remind me of my youth.

My college friends, Mike and Sal, have been a tremendous part of my support team. They flew to LA several times to be with me and keep my spirits up when Pamela took some weekend breaks and were always on the phone with me, and, since moving to San

Jose, they have been a tremendous part of my immediate support team.

And then there was a gift of immeasurable emotion from my friend, Gary. His mother had been fighting cancer for fifteen years and lost her battle in 2000. Always an outdoor person, she wanted to climb Mt. Everest someday, but cancer prevented her from attaining her goal. A friend of hers went to Tibet and obtained a *dorje*, which is a Tibetan artifact that represents the "thunderbolt of enlightenment," and is recognized as having healing and spiritual qualities. The friend carried the *dorje* to Mt. Everest and brought it back to Gary's mother. Gary's mother was told that her prognosis was poor and that she had only a few months to live. Upon receiving the *dorje*, she had it with her every day, finally losing her battle after almost two years later than predicted. Gary sent the *dorje* to me believing that it would give me hope. It did. I held it often, and it was always by my bedside.

Friends like these are of great support, especially when they give meaningful expressions of themselves that express the height of their generosity and love.

My friends were there for us in so many ways.

My brother-in-law, Kevin, and his wife, Linda, are deeply religious people. Kevin went through his own difficulties with substance abuse many years ago, and we were there to help him through it. When we needed him, he and Linda were there. They flew down to Los Angeles several times and prayed for and with us. Linda would go shopping and clean the house. They really were there for us whenever we needed them.

A very good friend, Patty, sent me a card every week for at least a year.

One of my chamber board members, Rod, sent me a portable DVD player so that Pamela and I could watch movies in bed when I was not isolated.

Another friend, Eric, who is a musician, cut CDs of his own music, which I played constantly in my room.

The employees of the chamber held their own blood drive and, as I have said, worked above and beyond the call of duty.

Pamela's friend from Sacramento, Ada, called her several times each day since the beginning of my illness to make sure she was OK. Those phone calls were a great source of strength.

A member of Congress from LA, Lucille Roybal-Allard, who had become a close friend, visited me several times and called Pamela to remain in touch.

Friends invited Pamela for dinner.

Tannis, a bone marrow transplant survivor from Australia was in town and spent time with me. We have since corresponded via e-mail, and she is a part of our support network.

Others went grocery shopping and stayed with Pamela to help her at night.

Our neighbors and friends, Tamara and Steve, constantly had Pamela over for dinner and helped her relax on difficult days.

Cards, calls, e-mails, and other communication ensured that I remained in touch with those closest to me.

## Friends Are for Life

When I first was diagnosed with leukemia, I did not know how things would turn out—where the road would lead. We were in a relatively new place, and, while we had a few friends, we were not living near any family or any of my lifetime friends. My brother, Mark, who lived in New Jersey, called me every day I was in the hospital. My brother, Lee, called often, and was my platelet donor at a moment's notice. Without him I would not have had the life-saving blood product I needed.

I soon learned that miles do not separate true friends. I spoke about Steve, Karen, and Sam. They made so many trips to LA during my treatments that I cannot even count them. They were at the hospital. They made gifts. They spent time at home with Pamela. They cared for her. They cared for me. Without them I do not know what I would have done.

During my ordeal I met two transplant survivors, Brian and Vicki, who had different experiences. Vicki returned to a more normal life within a few years and was running a marathon within five years. Brian had a harder course and it took him nearly ten years to return to a normal life at work. They were tremendous supporters at crucial times because they had walked the walk. They came to visit. They called me on the phone. They knew what I was going through and could empathize with me about the struggles and challenges I was facing. I could not have gone through the ups and downs without them and they remain a key part of my support team to this day.

Iris and Al have been friends for thirty years. Iris was with us the day of my transplant. They called and visited many times. They flew down from Sacramento and were of great support, especially for Pamela.

Three Los Angeles City council members, Eric Garcetti, Jan Perry, and Jack Weiss, immediately volunteered to give blood and be tested to see if they were marrow matches.

Suzanne, my former assistant from Sacramento, is a dear friend, and she also flew down to LA to be by my side. We had a great relationship as coworkers that continues today as friends.

Adrienne is a businesswoman I met in LA who was always checking in with me. She introduced me to a fellow patient who I talked with from time to time.

Mike and Lisa were neighbors from Sacramento who kept in constant touch with Pamela, which always made me feel at ease. They sent funny DVDs, cards, and anything that would make me laugh.

Ethel is the mother of a high school friend, and, although her husband was fighting his own illness at the time, she always sent cards, nearly each week.

Lori and Joe were good friends from San Jose who were another source of great comfort to Pamela, as were Sue and Darrell. Sue and Lori came down to be with Pamela on the day of my transplant.

I was involved in an organization in Sacramento called the American Leadership Forum that promotes collaborative leadership principles. I cannot say enough about the support I received from my ALF senior fellows, specifically my special buddy, Sally, and others including Doni, Dennis, Bev, Rick, Gina, Brenda, Don, Carol, Mario, Rick, Paula, Evelyn, and Marian.

In my years in the chamber of commerce business, I came to see it as a family. Executives came to know each other very personally and often rallied around each other. That was true in a big way during my illness. I could never list the hundreds of names of chamber executives who called and sent their best wishes to us, and still do. I would thank Dave Kilby and Mick Fleming who are the presidents of the Western Association of Chamber Executives and the American Chamber of Commerce Executives, respectively.

They kept the associations and the members aware of what was going on with me and are great friends.

I was blessed to have a great assistant in LA as well. Ellie did a great job keeping me plugged in while I was home and in the hospital and always called and visited to make sure we kept in touch. She even traveled with me to St. Louis for a conference to make sure I could go and be sworn in as chair-elect of the American Chamber of Commerce Executives.

Chris Martin and his wife, Jeannette, were very good friends. Chris was one of the chairs of the chamber, and they lived nearby. They were there to help us and kept in touch with Pamela.

I wrote about George Kieffer; he and his wife, Judith, were always supporters of us and always kept in touch with Pamela and the family. Somewhat fortuitously, Gerald got his first job working for Judith.

Matt Toledo is a great friend from LA, and he came to the hospital many times along with his daughters. He was always calling and, most importantly, he checked in on Pamela constantly.

I learned that true friends are there for life, and I hope that all of you who are friends to people in positions of need respond as mine did.

## Just being there is enough

In times of illness, people often do not know what to say to those in need. Often they ask questions like, "How can I help?" or "What do you need?" or "What can I do?" These are hard questions to answer because often there is little that others can do in a concrete way—except just being there.

When you reach out to a friend, I ask you to remember that, more often than not, just being there is enough. The little things do help. Make a phone call. Pay a visit. Send an e-mail. Write a card and personalize it. These contacts are often just what a sick person needs. I can't tell you how much the cards and letters meant to me. I received in excess of one thousand of them, and I received them constantly. I read them all but could not respond each one. I was simply overwhelmed. But they gave me great comfort. Pamela and I opened the mail together every day, and I cannot express the inspiration those messages brought to us.

One important thing: don't just be there at the height of the illness. Remember that patients with cancer often have a long recuperation and recovery. Don't forget about them when they leave the hospital. That is when they need you the most. Telephone calls, visits, notes, and e-mails do wonders. Remember that there will be long, lonely, and difficult days for a long time and stay in touch. My friends have done so for me, and they continue to do so to this day.

Here are some other things that can help:

- Ask if you can do research for the patient
- Start a prayer group
- Set up an e-mail list
- Bring meals for the patient or the family
- Offer to be a driver
- Send a masseuse
- Bring movies to the hospital or the home
- Send a housekeeper to the home from time to time

Here are some of the notes that kept me going. I thought I would include just a few samples of notes from some of these friends.

Rusty,

Good luck. Barbara and I simply wanted you to know we are thinking of you. We admire your spirit and wish we could help but maybe it does help in a tiny bit to know that your many friends are with you.

As you fight the good fight with all your might just know that a lot of folks are in your corner praying for you, admiring you, and loving you.
—President George H. W. Bush

I am so sorry to hear of your recent setbacks. I know that your courage will pull you thorough and that you will be back on top once again.
—Anonymous

Occasionally we have the opportunity to receive a gift that transcends the entire community. Through the blood and marrow drive done on your behalf, you, and your family has given Blood Source a very special gift. I express my sincere appreciation for your passion for people and for life. Please know that we stand ready to return your kindness to Blood Source and to the Sacramento community.
—Leslie Botos, Blood Source

I was so sorry to hear that you have been struck by this wretched disease and simply wanted to send a note to say how much I am thinking about you—and your family—during such a different time for all of you. Although I gather the treatment is rather tough I shall remain optimistic of its outcome.
—The Rt. Hon. John Major

I feel your pain and will add some prayers your way. I appreciate all you've done and feel "you the man"—like maybe there's more expected for you on this Earth—so hang in there and look for the best in all around you, and best wishes for your recovery.
—Anonymous

You will continue to be in our thoughts and prayers and we hope to see you cheering at a Kings game—even if it is in Los Angeles.
—Joe and Gavin Maloof, Owners, Sacramento Kings, NBA

Your tremendous energy is contagious and will get you through this
—Al/Iris

Keep your hands in God's ever loving hands and know that friends like me are with you.
—John Bryant

The physical pain Rusty has endured in fighting for his life is beyond human comprehension. He fights for his life

because he loves you, his children, and his family. When all of the material goodies of his life get stripped away, what remains is our spiritual and loving connection to each other that bonds each other to this life. The outpouring of love to Rusty just shows what esteem he holds. He is a great guy, who truly has a "wonderful life."
—Gino/Louise

I am thoroughly convinced that a positive mental outlook goes a long way toward defeating an enemy. I know you are a fighter and will ultimately win this battle. Just remember, don't ever, ever, ever quit.
—General H. Norman Schwarzkopf, Retired

Fight this thing with all you've got. We need you back.
—LA Chamber staff

This card cost me 2 stamps!
—Mike

Please accept this as a warm tribute to your guts and courage. Love and strength, my friend and brother.
—Chris Matthews

You have been courageous and inspiring as you deal with your illness and all of us who have witnessed your determination to overcome this disease are grateful for this example.
—Roger Cardinal Mahony

You have been an inspiration—not just in the courage and determination you have shown through your illness, but that you have shown your dedication to Los Angeles through this entire ordeal. I cannot think of anyone who would face a life threatening ordeal and would continue to think of his obligations to his employer and to his city at the same time. You are truly a jewel of our city.
—LA City Councilman Eric Garcetti

It's time to focus on your life, your love, and your family. You have given so much of yourself to your community and your work. It's now time to give back to yourself. It is an honor knowing you and working with you. Kick Cancer's Ass!
—Marlee Miller

I wanted to drop a note to wish you the best of luck and pray for your good health and to thank you for all you have done to help me improve our education system. You are a true leader for children in our state and I look forward to working with you when you are back on top.
—Rob Reiner

I'm very sorry to learn that you're stepping down as president of the Los Angeles Area Chamber of Commerce. You've done a great job as our chamber's leader. Rusty, I wish you all the best as you take some time off to recover your health. You are in our thoughts and prayers.
—Steven B. Sample, President, USC

Rusty, you are showing tremendous courage in your fight and we are so lucky that you are continuing to work with us while you are ill. Having you as our CEO at less than fifty percent is better than having someone full time, so just know that we will always support you and work with you.
—Chris Martin, Chamber Vice Chair

A little bird that goes around spreading news tweeted to me that you are having a rough time of it. I just wanted you to know that I am among your scores of friends who are wishing you a speedy recovery and will be closely following your progress back to good health
—Walter Cronkite

*That's What Friends Are For*[32]

Knowin' you can always count on me, for sure
That's what friends are for.
—Stevie Wonder

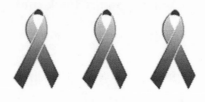

---

32  http://www.lyrics007.com/Stevie%20Wonder%20Lyrics/That's%20What%20Frie nds%20Are%20For%20Lyrics.html

# CHAPTER 6

# SUGGESTIONS TO IMPROVE MEDICAL CARE

I certainly lived through many experiences that taught me many things about how the medical community could improve its services to patients. Here are some ideas that I hope they will consider.

I am not an expert in health care, but I have learned a lot about it over the last several years. From being in six hospitals and working with over fifty physicians, perhaps double that number of nurses, and hundreds of technicians, social workers, and other hospital staff from administrators to maintenance staff, I have many observations about the patient/medical care relationship.

Practicing medicine is one of the most difficult pursuits that can be undertaken by a man or woman. Doctors deal with the most complex object on Earth: the human body. They speak in languages and concepts that are difficult to master, let alone be understood by those of us who do not have a medical background. They sacrifice their lives for years in school and residencies and more advanced education. They hold the lives of their patients in their hands. They save lives every day, and when their efforts are not enough, they often find themselves in court defending their actions. They are always on duty and must always be ready for dealing with the most complex of human problems—both physical and emotional. They live in a world full of regulations that affect what they can and cannot do, who they can and cannot talk to, and what they can and cannot say. Being a doctor is one of life's most rewarding endeavors, yet it can be one of the most stressful ones, and I have the greatest respect for those who enter the profession.

But also, as can any professional in any given field, doctors (and indeed the entire health care community) can learn something from the rest of us. They can learn from patients. They can learn from caregivers, family members, and all who come into contact with them.

I will begin by showing health care as a continuing loop rather than a hierarchy of caregivers. My diagram of the way we should think of the relationships is shown below. I call it The Healing Circle. It is a simple concept, one that we think happens every day. Then, I will present some lessons I wish medical providers would learn, or commonsense suggestions that I believe would improve patient care, especially in the face of a life-threatening illness.

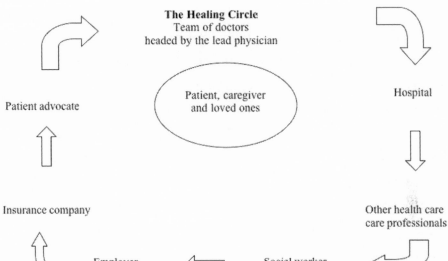

Patient advocate

Insurance company

Employer

Social worker

Hospital

Other health care
care professionals

1. The patient and his or her loved ones are at the center of the circle. That sounds like a given but in my experience it does not always happen that way. All too often, doctors see themselves at the center with the world revolving around them. Things are done at the whim and convenience of the physician. Decisions may be made without consulting the patient in advance. I believe that doctors must reorient themselves to believing and acting like the patient is at the center of the universe and that the patient is in control of his or her destiny. To do this, they could do the following:

   a. Communicate clearly, effectively, and in terms the patient can understand. Remember PHRASE.

   b. Make sure the patient understands what is being said before the encounter with the patient is over.

   c. Consult with the patient about when and where tests will be taken to make sure the patient is ready physically and emotionally.

   d. Communicate with the families. All too often, I have been in bed with my wife by my side and the physician acted like she was not there and would respond to her questions by looking at me. The role of the family in the wellness of the patient cannot be minimized.

   e. Communicate more effectively among themselves. I have firsthand experience of doctors prescribing medications that conflict, ordering duplicate tests, or giving conflicting advice. This only unnecessarily confuses the patient and his or her family and could be easily avoided if the physicians looked at themselves as a part of a patient team rather than individual specialists.

f.  Listen to what the patient has to say. Doctors must listen to the person laying in the bed as an individual and recognize that they have specific needs that must be addressed that may be outside of protocols or may differ from what the physician may normally tend to prescribe in any given situation.

In one example that impacted my wellness, I asked a physician to refer me to the pain management specialists because my pain was getting out of control. While I knew that my doctor was doing the best he could to ease my pain, it just was not working. Was he using the right medication? Could something else be used in combination with what I was taking to bring a more effective result? This particular doctor pooh-poohed the specialty of pain management and indicated that he could control my pain. Only after nearly a week of my insisting on a referral to pain management did he call in the specialists. And they made a big difference.

2.  Patients must be at the top of their game emotionally if they are to survive physically. That means that social workers play a key role in patient wellness. Unfortunately, the social service programs I have seen in the six hospitals I have occupied have generally been below par, in my judgment. The social worker usually visits the patient upon admission and asks him or her

to fill out a simple form to indicate the level of stress the patient has—whether the stress was about finances, work, family, death, etc. Then they repeat the exercise before discharge. At least in my case, there was seldom any follow-up on what I said in my questionnaire to help me deal with the issues. The social workers were all nice people but, sadly, I felt alone in dealing with the many issues with which critically ill patients must cope.

The emotional recovery takes years longer than the physical. Programs are needed to help long-term survivors recover. Psychologists and social workers without BMT experience just don't get it.[33] Transplant Recipient—1996

The health care community must stress the importance of patient mental health to the healing process and provide the benefits and services to help patients as much mentally as they do physically.

3.  Hospitals must condition their employees to think of patients first. I cannot tell you how many times I was awakened in the middle of the night by an attendant who had come into my room to empty a urinal and turned on all of the room lights and flushed the toilet with the bathroom door wide open. I wondered, had he or she ever heard of flashlights? Of closing the

---

33  Fred Hutchinson Cancer Research Center. Long Term Follow Up Program, *Thoughts and Comments from Patients*

door? What about waiting until morning? It is hard enough for patients to sleep at night without unnecessary interruptions.

This brings me to the constant through-the-night wake up routine during which staff took my temperature and blood pressure. It is important to do that when a patient is critical. But if the patient is not critical, medical providers should look at procedures and protocols and be flexible so that patients can get the overnight rest they need.

From an administrative standpoint, hospitals need to find ways to reduce the paperwork that patients must deal with. I have been admitted to the same hospitals multiple times, and every time, I needed to fill out the same paperwork. Even transfers from one unit to another during the same hospital admission required additional paperwork and signatures. The paper flow needs to be streamlined so that patients and their families are not continually filling out the same forms and answering the same questions in the same ways inordinate numbers of times.

4. Other health care professionals play a critical role in patient recovery as well. They, too, must readjust their thinking to place patient comfort and convenience over departmental schedules. If a patient is just not ready for yet another test that day, staff members who are in charge of maintaining schedules should postpone the test unless the test is to diagnose a life-threatening condition.

I have the utmost respect for nurses. Throughout my ordeal, I developed a new understanding of the role nurses play. They are with us patients around the clock. They must have a detailed knowledge of the medical procedures, medications, signs, and symptoms of patient distress. All in all, nurses do a remarkable job, but they are often caught up in the schedule game, patient overload, and administrative duties. Nurses must be freed up to provide the quality of care that each patient needs.

5.  Although we don't normally think about it, I include the patient's employer as a part of the health care system. Going back to the mental health of the patient, one of the key stresses a patient undergoes is a worry about his or her job and, as a result, about financial issues. Employers need to be in the loop in the event that one of their employees becomes seriously ill; it is important that the patient and his or her family understand what the employer can and cannot do relative to keeping the patient's job open, what benefits are available, etc.

    More than that, I call upon the employment community to rethink its policies about employee illness. While it is normal to provide sick leave (usually ten to twelve days per year), which covers most people for casual illness, such allowances do not even come close to dealing with catastrophic cases. I urge employers to develop catastrophic illness policies to make sure employees are covered and that there are no gaps between sick leave and short-term and long-term disability benefits.

And, I remind employers that the best thing they can do with an ill employee is to stay in contact and keep the communication lines open, as the chamber did—especially if they need to fill the patient's position. The worst thing an employer can do is to shut down communication and leave the employee up in the air. Easing a patient's mental burden will speed his or her physical recovery.

6.  In addition to thinking about mental health, the medical community must think about physical conditioning—that means more than periodic physical therapy. It means gyms for patients, exercise counselors, and others who can work with patients to make sure that they focus on physical health to the best of their ability.

7.  The medical community must also understand the key role played by caregivers. Once patients leave the hospital after a major illness, they will generally need to rely on a caregiver to assist them with daily tasks. Unless the caregiver is a health care professional, sending the patient home without training the caregiver or providing support groups to help the caregiver cope and be effective, is like casting them on the water without sailing lessons.

8.  Insurance companies are a part of the game as well and must understand that they must be an active part of making things

easy on patients. They must pay bills on time. They should not delay prior authorizations or delay approvals for medications and procedures that are needed. At the bottom line, whether a patient needs something must be a decision made between him or her and the physician, and managed care should not unnecessarily interfere.

In addition, insurance companies need to make sure that mental health care is included in benefits because, for cancer patients, these services are just as critical as physical and medical care.

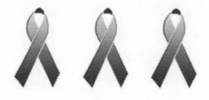

# CHAPTER 7

# IF YOU ARE RECOVERING FROM CANCER

Since day one, I focused on recovery. There is no day that recovery begins, and there is no day that it ends. Recovery is an ongoing process, and as much as does treatment, recovery takes great determination and courage. I received that determination from the words of a popular song which gave me reason to look forward.

*What a Wonderful World*[34]

I see trees of green, red roses too ...
And I think to myself, what a wonderful world.
—Louis Armstrong

This, one of my favorite songs, speaks to me about generational change, about renewal; about all of the things that make our world go around. The words always give me hope that as each day dawns,

---

34   http://www.lyricsfreak.com/l/louis+armstrong/what+a+wonderful+world_
     20085347.html

there will be new roses that bloom, new trees that reach toward the skies, and people reaching toward their ambitions and seek out their goals. It is the ability to embrace the small but profound beauties life has to offer that motivate and stimulate people like me who face life-threatening crises to recover and to once again rise up and use their talents.

Recovery means different things to different people. Some patients expect that they will recover to the normal levels of function that they had before they became ill. Still others hope just to be alive. And others have no idea what to expect. How a patient feels about his or her recovery is all about expectations.

I spoke recently with a cancer survivor who related the following conversation with his doctor several weeks after surgery to remove a tumor in his mouth:

> Doctor: Well, Harvey (alias), it looks like the surgery was a success.
>
> Harvey: Do you think you got all of the cancer?
>
> Doctor: Yes, we think we did—and best of all, you are alive.
>
> Harvey: But I am always in pain and have a hard time eating. I don't really enjoy my life these days. When will things get better?
>
> Doctor: We don't know for sure, but you are alive.
>
> Harvey: Am I? What is my quality of life?

Clearly, Harvey's expectations were not met.

Harvey's is a common reaction. The doctors are focused on curing the cancer and not as much as I believe they should be on quality of life through recovery. How will the patient respond to the treatment? What health problems will be ongoing? What side effects will dominate the patient's future life?

I do not mean, in any way, to alarm you. But I must be realistic in helping you prepare for recovery and recuperation by telling you that it may not be a bed of roses for you.

It may be replete with challenges. Or it may be easy. The only way to prepare for your recovery is to realize that there is no way to predict what it will be like.

I can understand that Harvey was feeling like he'd almost rather have not have not survived because I have felt same despair first-hand. (Sadly, as this book was going to press, Harvey passed away). There were many days at the City of Hope when I would see other patients, like me, seemingly ghosts walking aimlessly, looking for help, for relief, for hope.

I am a living example that, in many cases, the treatment can be worse than the disease. The doctors did their job by saving my life—they took me into remission so that I could live longer. But often there is not as much active thought as to the quality of life the patient will have post-transplant.

I have talked with many patients who came away from the experience with considerable side effects and post-transplant issues that were largely unresolved and would leave them ill for years to come.

If I had known prior to the transplant how poor my quality of life would be, I would not have had the procedure. I hate how I

feel, look, and act. I feel like I'm a lot worse off than before the
transplant.

Allogeneic transplant recipient—2003[35]

And yet, there are others who do very well with their transplant
and go on to live productive, long lives.

In July I will celebrate the 30th anniversary of my BMT.
I feel very fortunate that I have my good health and that my transplant has given me these 30 years to live life.

Allogeneic transplant recipient—1974[36]

There is no way to know going in. It is a hard choice to make,
and doctors must be more forthright in discussing side effects and
complications with patients in advance so that they can make clear
decisions.

There are many elements to recovery; it is not just physical
recovery. Emotional recovery, taking control of your life, picking
up the pieces, regaining hope for the future, dreaming new dreams,
repairing relationships, gaining energy for new endeavors, and trying to return to a more normal existence in the face of tremendous
uncertainty and new restrictions on your physical abilities are all
aspects of recuperation with which patients and caregivers must
cope. Another transplant survivor said:

---

35   Fred Hutchinson Cancer Research Center. Long Term Follow Up Program,
     *Thoughts and Comments from Patients.*
36   Ibid.

I try and fold as much into my life as I can. The last four years
have really been a roller coaster. There have been times where I've
felt pretty good and I've acquired a lot of responsibilities, and
then gotten sick and had to give those up. But all of those desires
still remain, definitely, and hope that one day those things will
return is part of what drives me. I think hope is what drives us
all. Hope is definitely what drives me. Without hope, what do you
have?[37]

—Transplant survivor

Perhaps the best way to think of recovery and reentry is in the
context of people who have served in the military or who have
been exposed to disasters like the destruction of the World Trade
Center. Having been exposed to severe trauma, their diagnosis is
often referred to as post-traumatic stress disorder.

Many of us have read about post-traumatic stress disorder
(PTSD) that can occur following the experience or witnessing of
life-threatening events such as military combat, natural disasters,
terrorist incidents, serious accidents, or violent personal assaults
and crime. People who suffer from it often relive the experience
through nightmares and flashbacks, have difficulty sleeping, and
feel detached or estranged, and these symptoms can be severe
enough and last long enough to significantly impair the person's
daily life.

---

37   Ibid.

I submit that going through life-threatening experiences, like cancer, is as traumatic as witnessing life-threatening events, and people need to be treated much like these stress victims. It is all a part of smoothing their recovery and reentry to as normal a life as is possible.

For me, I can't say when the recovery phase began; if I really think about it, I should say it began on the day I started treatment. On that day, I decided that this disease would not take me and that I would apply all of my will and courage to survival. Should this disease someday take my life, I do not want anyone to say—or for me to think at the end—that there was something I could have done in a reasonable way to keep on going and to preserve my life in a quality way.

Recovery and reentry are not easy. In my case, the hospital was my home for most of the first year. Since this ordeal began, I have spent more time in hospitals than I have in my own home. As of the completion of this book, the longest consecutive period of time I have been out of the hospital has been three months. As my "home," the hospital provided me security. People were there to help whenever I needed anything. I made many friends among the staff. Everything in the hospital became familiar. My hospital family—my fellow patients, our loved ones, and the staff talked, we joked, we cried, and we shared our experiences. It was my security blanket. Leaving the protective womb of the hospital was not easy. Nor was it free of emotion.

And once I headed for home after the transplant hopefully for a very long time—I knew that staying positive and doing everything I should to facilitate the best recovery I could, would take a new level of discipline. I would need to depend on Pamela to care for me. I would need to be responsible for my own medications, itself a major task as I was taking up to forty medications daily. It would not be easy. To survive this mentally as well as physically, I would need to focus on being well, dealing with medications, getting exercise, and having a positive mental attitude.

But a positive recovery requires more than just focus especially if you are going home after an extended time away. In that event, remember that you are no longer a part of the normal routine around your household. Things may have been moved to different places. Household members may have new habits. Pets may not remember you. You must take these changes in stride, recognizing that you need to ease back into your surroundings.

In addition, you will find that your duties may have been taken on by others. This can lead to feeling that you are no longer needed or useful to your family.

You will find that you just cannot do things that you were able to do before cancer. Your energy will likely be low, and just getting up to get a drink will be a chore. You will tire easily. Preparing a meal may be out of the question. This will be frustrating, but it will get better.

You must also be prepared, and prepare your partner if you have one, to deal with the fact that you may not have the energy, capacity, or interest in intimacy for some time. Partly, this will be due to your lack of energy. Partly, it may simply be an effect of the treatment. Be prepared. Talk about it honestly. You will find that your love will get you through even though you may be physically, mentally, or emotionally limited.

From a wellness perspective, some ideas that can help you once you are home:

- <u>Make sure the house is well cleaned.</u>

  Your biggest enemy is germs, so you must obsess over cleanliness.

- <u>Eat as much as you can.</u>

  You need fuel for energy, even though you will be on a limited diet.

  Your nutrition needs will vary. A nutritionist can help you develop a proper and balanced diet that will help you maintain and promote your overall health. These will include the following:

  - Proteins to ensure growth, to repair body tissue, and to maintain a healthy immune system. Without enough protein, the body takes longer to recover from illness and lowers resistance to infection. Good sources of protein include lean meat, fish, poultry, dairy products, nuts, dried beans, peas and lentils, and soy foods.

  - Vitamins and minerals will promote proper growth and development.

  - Carbohydrates include fruits, vegetables, breads, pasta, grains and cereal products, dried beans, peas, and lentils. Sources of fat include butter; margarine; oils; nuts; seeds; and the fat in meats, fish, and poultry. Carbohydrates and fats supply most of the calories you will need.

  - Water and fluids are necessities to avoid dehydration— a slippery slope you do not want to have to reverse.

- <u>Exercise</u>.

  The sooner you start to walk, the better you'll eventually feel. You'll find that, in the first few days of leaving the hospital, you will be more fatigued than you've ever been in your life. That's normal, but once again you have to try and push yourself and even have your caregiver push you to do some exercise. On my first day home, I walked for five minutes and felt like collapsing. Don't over-exceed your limits. You'll quickly find that your stamina improves and your general energy levels increase as you build up your walks.

- <u>Wash your hands regularly</u>.

  Avoid touching your mouth and nose. Your hands pick up much dirt and grime easily, and you can transfer that to your face if not careful and get an infection.

- <u>Avoid crowds</u>.

  If you must be in a crowd, wear a mask to prevent the spread of germs.

- <u>Avoid the sun</u>.

  Use the strongest sun block on exposed skin when in the sun. You will probably find that many of you medications are not compatible with sun exposures.

- <u>Set mini goals for yourself</u>.

  The goals can be as simple as driving the car or cooking your own meal or making something. Suddenly ordinary everyday tasks will become really fun and help you to feel more normal.

- <u>Don't become isolated</u>.

  Yes, you are sick, but you are not in prison. Make sure you stay in contact with friends. Encourage them to visit. If you have the stamina, visit them; but remember, you have a long way to go until you will be as able to travel as you were before the transplant.

- <u>Keep writing in your diary</u>.

  You will wish you had a detailed record of your treatments, medications, visitors, feelings, and observations. I had some notes but now wish I had more.

- <u>Stay away from anyone who is ill.</u>

  This is especially true of young children who have been exposed to or anyone who has received a live virus or vaccine.

My recovery came in two phases. The first was the recovery from the chemo, radiation, and transplant. The second was the recovery from the complications of the treatment—specifically the osteoporosis, broken hip, fractures, and related issues. My recovery from these two phases is ongoing.

At least I thought that these were the two phases of my recovery.

At the end of June 2006, I entered the third phase of my recovery—my emotional recovery. I officially retired as president and CEO of the LA Chamber. Cleaning out my office and saying goodbye to my dedicated group of employees was difficult and emotional. As I told them, it was tough leaving a job you love, knowing that you can do the job mentally but not physically.

It brought back the realization that I continued to live in limbo. There was no way to predict, from one day to another, what the day would be like. How would I feel? What would I be able to do?

I continue to struggle with the changing roles between Pamela and me. Whereas I was always the breadwinner and was able to effectively provide for the family, I can no longer do so, and we live off a disability check, which in no way equals anything close to my prior compensation. We used to share the household duties. I loved to cook and now can do little of that anymore. I just do not have the strength or stamina. It is just so hard to watch her shoulder the burdens of our everyday life.

But I know that these are the realities of my disease and I/we are dealing with them the best we can. It is just that the future is so uncertain.

I know that the numbers are not in my favor and that I will always run the risk of a recurrence and a less than desirable quality of life, but I also know that I will live every day to its fullest. I know that I have some serious issues to deal with that are the result of the leukemia and its treatment. I will, in many respects, be fighting these for the rest of my life.

This disease has changed my life in so many ways. Despite the uncertainty, I must redefine my life on new terms, with new limits to my role as a provider, husband, and father.

I cannot surrender to leukemia or its complications. I need to keep on going.

I need to keep on going because I must be there to see the weddings of my children and the births of my grandchildren.

I need to keep going because my wife and I are just getting to know each other after thirty years of marriage, and we have so much more to do together—so many more hours, days, weeks, months, and years of love left.

I need to keep on going so that others can see how one can positively respond when cancer calls.

I really do not know how to answer the question: Would I do it again if I had the same choice? I think at first glance I would say yes, because you always say yes to life. That is the natural reaction. But in my case, I have been dealt a poor deck of cards. My quality of life has given me so many second thoughts that it is not an easy answer. The list of disabilities I am and will be saddled with clearly shows that, while we have defeated leukemia for now, the side effects and aftereffects of the disease and medications are heavy burdens I will carry with me forever. So in my case, the treatment has clearly been a difficult course.

There is no way the doctors could have laid out for me that I would have developed the co-morbidities that I have developed, because everyone responds differently to treatments and medications. That is why I have said throughout this book that you should not be frightened to undergo treatment based simply upon how it has impacted me. The way the treatment has impacted me if just that—the way it has impacted me. Many other people have come through it just fine. But in my case whether to go through it again if I knew I would have the exact same result would be a tough choice. If there had been a time machine that could have laid out specifically all of the side effects and aftereffects that I have had to contend with, I must say that the choice would not be easy or obvious. I certainly have lived each day I have been given and am thankful for that. I am thankful for every day I have had with my wife, children, family, friends, loved ones, and others. I have taken full advantage of writing this book to put my thoughts, ideas, and philosophy down for posterity. But there have been days when the pain and burden have been just too much. These are not easy choices.

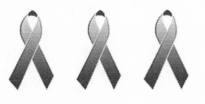

# PART III

# REFLECTIONS

# CHAPTER 8

# FOR MY PAMELA

*Have I Told You Lately?*[38]

Fill my heart with gladness
Ease my troubles, that's what you do.
—Rod Stewart

As I have said in other parts of this book, my wife, Pamela, is the most important person in my life and has been by my side for over thirty years. She is, in many respects, the reason that I was able to survive my treatment to this time and to write this book. She has been my inspiration and my rock throughout. I could not have done it without her.

There is little I can teach Pamela; she has taught me more than I could ever impart to her. I hope that I have shown her that our love and our relationship are for a lifetime; she certainly has shown me that. When in a position facing death, you always wonder whether

---

38  http://www.lyrics007.com/Rod%20Stewart%20Lyrics/Have%20I%20Told%20Yo
u%20Lately%20Lyrics.html

you have told your spouse or the ones you love how you feel about them. Rod Stewart's words say it much better than I ever could.

During one especially difficult time in my treatment, in the long, dark, and lonely hours, I decided to put pen to paper and write a poem to Pamela that I showed her only when she read the draft of this book:

## I Will Never Leave You

I am engaged in the battle for my life;
You have been there with me every step of the way.

I have the will to be with you forever;
I just hope my body will cooperate.

But if I lose this battle before it is my time,
Know that I will never leave you

I may not be there to hold or embrace you,
But my love and spirit will follow you always.

So if tomorrow finds us forever apart in this world,
Keep me with you always in my heart.

And have faith that we will someday
Be together again.

Pamela and I have shared some incredibly happy years. From having traveled to wonderful places around the world to having our beautiful children to meeting famous people and having wonderful friends and homes, it has been a wonderful life. Our struggles have been few.

But like all couples, we have experienced our ups and downs. There is no shame in that. Our feelings for each other and the strength of our marriage held us together through these tough times, only to find us in the position of this horrible disease. During this entire time, Pamela has been the model partner and, in a strange way, this ordeal has strengthened our relationship.

I cannot tell you how much agony I felt as I saw the impact of my illness on Pamela. To see her every day going through the pain of the journey broke my heart. To hold her hand as we rushed to the intensive care unit not once, but several times, was agonizing. To see her standing in a dark hallway in the middle of the night as I was taken for a CT scan after a fall or to rule out a brain bleed, was a horrible sight to see. These experiences almost broke me.

The pain was beyond measure.

We have been fortunate that in the thirty years since we committed to each other on a sunny summer day in a beautiful garden setting, we meant that commitment to last forever.

As we move forward, there is no way to predict the future. I have good days and bad days. I never know when I will be home or back in the hospital. I cannot know the struggles and loneliness Pamela faces when I sleep for hours during the day or cannot be around her. I pray for her always.

Most importantly, I want her to take care of herself. That is hard to do when she is so wrapped up in my care, but it is so vital. I have been fortunate in that Pamela has been there every day for me. I have seen so many patients who find themselves alone at best, or neglected at worst. Not me. I could not pry Pamela away from the hospital. I could not convince her to leave.

And I must tell her and any spouse that taking care of a cancer patient is a huge relief to the patient. I, for one, knew that I would be taken care of in the hospital. But what I never knew was who would take care of Pamela, who would walk her to the car, hold her hand, and give her a shoulder to cry on, who would help around the house and take care of her when I could not. The distress this gave me was immense.

From a day-to-day standpoint, my illness has been difficult on her in many other ways. This applies to the day-to-day chores and to aspects of her daily life as well. Pamela has had to sacrifice her career. She has given up any social life or "normal life" with a healthy partner. She has sacrificed her life and given up a great deal of her identity. She has shown that she has an astounding source of strength.

I have tried to put my game face on for her as well. On days when I just did not feel up to seeing her, I would pick myself up and be the best I could be. I would do my best to mask the pain or discomfort. If I was drowsy from the medications, I would do whatever I could to stay awake. I would always ask her to lay down in bed with me. I would try my best to nurture her.

These were my ways of being a caregiver for her.

But it is also critical for caregivers to take care of themselves.

So I say to her and to spouses that we, as patients, want you to take care of yourselves.

And if the outcome of our battle ends prematurely and not the one we'd hoped for, please take care of yourself when we can no longer do so. Knowing that you will do so will be of great relief and comfort to us.

And I know that, on my last of days, I will sing these words to Pamela:

*One More Day*[39]

One more sunset maybe I'd be satisfied …
Leave me wishing still, for one more day with you.
—Diamond Rio

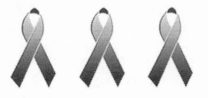

---

39   http://www.lyrics007.com/Diamond%20Rio%20Lyrics/One%20More%20Day%20Lyrics.html

# CHAPTER 9

# MY ETHICAL LEGACY

When I first decided to write this book, I decided that a central element of why I was doing it was so that I could leave something to my children that would help them guide their lives. I did not know whether leukemia would claim me before I'd had the opportunity to teach them the life lessons that they can use to shape their future. The more I thought about it, the more I realized that this legacy could be used by others as they looked to moral and ethical guideposts from a person who had lived a good life that might be cut short. Who else has the gift of time to give to others than someone like me who has the time and acuity to think about and record beliefs for posterity? So while I don't mean to be preachy, I hope that others can use these thoughts as they choose to shape their lives and their own legacies.

Leaving an ethical legacy is my way of communicating what I believe to be the essential characteristics that are important to living a productive and valued life. Central to that is making the commitment to never taking life for granted; making the most out of every opportunity. Lee Ann Womack put my sentiments to music in the following song:

*I Hope You Dance*[40]

And when you get the choice to sit it out or dance,
I hope you dance.
—Lee Ann Womack

The full lyrics of Womack's song tell young people to always strive for adventure and "never lose the hunger," to love, to have faith, to never settle for the easy way out, to take charge of their lives, to never sell out, and most of all to engage in something when they have a chance—to not sit life out.

These are the sentiments that are at the heart of my ethical legacy; it is based on my desire for young people to engage their lives and make them worthwhile for themselves, for their children, and for the future of their communities and their fellow citizens. Jewish tradition speaks of the notion of an ethical will, something I was briefly introduced to briefly by Bruce Feldstein, MD, and D'vorah Rose, RN, of the Jewish Chaplaincy Service at Stanford Hospital. Both have become close friends and confidants during my journey.

When confronted with death, I was overcome with how I lived my life. What had I accomplished? Would my presence on Earth be remembered? Had it been a life worth living?

---

40　http://www.lyrics007.com/Lee%20Ann%20Womack%20Lyrics/I%20Hope%20You%20Dance%20Lyrics.html

I soon realized that the best measure of whether I had lived a life worth living was in what I would pass on—to my children, to my wife, and to my friends. Such introspection forces you to think about what is important in life—to make sure that the guideposts and values under which you lived your life will be passed on. I hope you will understand these things and apply them in your lives.

My illness was, and remains to be, a difficult experience, and I do not know why I was called to bear this burden. But one thing I know is that it gave me the opportunity to teach my children lessons about life and courage and how to summon strength from within to battle the most difficult challenges that life can present.

To Gerald and Jennifer, and to all those who may read this book, these words tell you that you need to embrace life, take chances, and make life the best it can be for you. You never know what turns your life will take, where it will lead, what tomorrow will bring, or whether there will even be tomorrow. Live your life so that you can say that you lived it fully.

Here are some things that I think are essential to living a good and rewarding life. When I say rewarding, I do not mean in the sense of financial rewards for you. I mean it in the broadest sense of producing rewards for you and for others.

These are in no particular order of priority or necessity. That is the beauty of it, I believe. Take these lessons and apply them to your life in the priority and manner you choose; you can reject them all and develop your own code. In any event, think through these important issues and mold your life accordingly, not randomly.

I am not a philosopher. Nor am I a moralist. I am a person, just like you, striving to make the best out of every day of life that I am given, and I hope that these thoughts help you do the same. The words I chose for this section are among the most important ones that I have written, and I hope you will remember them.

## A full life is determined by how well you live.

We are all given time on this Earth, but it is just time. Everyone is given time; some use it more productively than others. We do not know how much time we are given. The amount of time can be long or it can be short. We never know when it will end; therefore, we must make the best use of every day we are given. God gives us skills, talent, intellect, and other capabilities, but it is up to us to decide what to do with them. This time we are given is a gift. The people we meet, the people we love, the places we visit, and the jobs we hold are all gifts that we must use wisely.

Just as we move into the prime times of our lives, we begin to near the end of our lives. But that is the hand we are dealt. As much as anyone, I have learned that we never know how much time we have left. So it is our duty to make our lives the best that they can be.

One person can make a difference. You owe all you come into contact with the best that you can give them. You owe your community, state, and country the benefit of all of your talents and expertise. Be a part of solving problems, not complaining about them. You know from my background that I believe you have an obligation to make the world a better place than you found it. You should live your life so others will say the world is a better place because you passed this way.

## A strong code of ethics is as reliable as a compass.

You have been raised to be ethical people. Integrity, honesty, reliability, and many other factors make up your own code of ethics, and you will build on them in the years ahead. If you follow these ethical guidelines, you will find that they will give you the answers you need to dilemmas that you will face when called upon to make tough decisions. You should, as we have tried to teach you, do unto others as you would have them do unto you. You should practice your moral and ethical behavior in that way, and it will come around back to you in just that way. Many decisions may appear difficult, but if you place them in the context of your code of ethics, the code will guide you to making the right decision.

> Real integrity is doing the right thing, knowing that nobody's
> going to know whether you did it or not.[41]
> Oprah Winfrey

## Be morally courageous.

Courage is something to be admired—but not just the physical courage of running into a burning building or fighting in a war. I am talking about moral courage: doing what is right despite the consequences. This could be blowing the whistle on corruption or speaking out against injustice or risking your situation by telling the truth.

---

41  http://www.quotationspage.com/quote/27014.html

It is curious that physical courage should be so common
in the world and moral courage so rare.[42]
Mark Twain

Martin Luther King Jr. had moral courage. Our founding fathers
had it. But history is littered with those who faced moral decisions
and did not show courage and paid a dear price for the lack of courage. Many of them may have been good people who were caught
up in a moral situation and decided to keep quiet rather than show
courage to stop what they knew was wrong. The world, now more
than ever, needs a generation of young people who need to stand
up and show moral and ethical courage in the face of injustice
around the world—who see the injustice of hunger, ethnic cleans-
ing, terrorism, and the many ills that plague our planet and say
that enough is enough; it is time that we reclaim ourselves and our
right to a decent life for all here on Earth.

So I urge you to recognize situations where morality is involved,
and show the courage of your morality to do what is right.

### Lead by example.

The best way to get people to work with and for you is to set a good
example. The old adage says, do as I do, not as I say. If you show a
positive example people will follow the example you set. If you are
negative, lazy, not creative, averse to risk, tardy, or condescending,
then others will be as well. So set a positive example; people will
follow your leadership.

---

42   http://www.quotationspage.com/quote/1985.html

## **<u>Trust is the single most important factor in personal and professional relationships.</u>**

Remember that your word is all you have. When you give your word, people must be able to trust in you. This is true of your personal life and your business life. Without people trusting in you to say what you mean, mean what you say, and keep your commitments, you will not be taken seriously by others.

## **<u>Promote justice for everyone.</u>**

There is injustice in our own country and around the world. Yet if each of us in our own way fights injustice we can make a difference to make sure that our rights are protected. Nothing is worse than seeing expressions of people's rights being trampled on or losing their liberties. Too many people have lost their lives or their own liberties fighting to protect the rights of others.

> Injustice anywhere is a threat to justice everywhere.
> Martin Luther King Jr.[43]

## **<u>Treat others as you would like to be treated.</u>**

Do unto others as you would have done unto yourself. What goes around comes around. How many times have you heard these expressions? But they are true. If you treat other people in the manner that you would like to be treated—and if I know you, that will be with care, compassion, and love—you will find that they will be there for you in the same way.

---

43   Letter from Birmingham Jail

## Teach and learn, forever.

Every day gives us the opportunity to learn, not only about facts but about life as well. Do not think that you have finished learning just because you have completed your formal education. Over your lifetime, you will learn from others—employers, friends, neighbors, and people you meet. Learn from them, apply those lessons to your life, and, most importantly, pass on what you have learned to others.

## Be humble.

Never be too full of yourself. You know that I had success early in life in my political career and have led a very public life. But I have always been uncomfortable taking credit for things in which I have been involved, whether in the community or at work. Showing humility is an important ingredient in focusing people and yourself on the outcomes of what you and others do, rather than seeking and taking credit and placing that above the importance of the results.

## Be an inspiration to others.

We can all serve as a role model to someone, and you should seek to be one. It could be to a child, a coworker, a friend, or anyone. You owe it to those who have not been as fortunate as you have been to show them ways of living and behaving that allow them to make the most out of their lives.

## Love each other—unconditionally.

If there is one thing we have tried to teach you, it is that love is the centerpiece of life. We have nothing if we do not have love. Our lives are empty without love. Love is as important as air, for it fulfills your life. It is the foundation on which families are built. So I ask you to always look to each other for love. I remind you that the bonds that tie you together as brother and sister—and more importantly as two human beings who have been together as twins since your time began—can never be broken and that it is your responsibility to keep our family together through bonds of love. As you grow translate that love to your families and see to it that your families are close. Remember, some day, when your mother and I are gone, you will be the heads of our family. Prepare for it by building a foundation of love.

Do not place conditions on your love for each other. One of you may disappoint the other at some time or do something that the other may disagree with. But always remember that we are all our own people and can make decisions about what to do and how to do it, but that nothing should ever interfere with the love you feel for each other.

## Stay close to each other.

As much as you need to love each other, I learned since my youth that a price is to be paid if families do not stay close. In our busy world, it is easy to lose touch, but that is a slippery slope to becoming alone and isolated. So please stay close together; keep your families close in the years ahead, and always find ways to be together.

## Keep your promises.

You are only as good as your word. You must be able to be trusted by all you come into contact with. Keep your promises and commitments so that you can be trusted.

## Always look for the best in people.

It is easy to be critical of others, but everyone has qualities that contribute to our society and to our understanding and growth. Everyone can make a contribution to our society; some make large contributions in the glare of the public while others toil in anonymity doing good works every day. But a gentle and kind person always looks for the best in people and finds ways to help that person accentuate their strengths.

## Find your soul mate in life, and don't settle.

If you are as lucky as I was and find someone as wonderful for yourself as your mother was for me, you will find true happiness. Find someone who places a premium on kindness, fairness, and developing shared goals for your future together. If you are that lucky, never have fear. You will never be alone. You will always be loved. As Berthold Brecht said, "Do not fear death so much, but rather the inadequate life."[44]

I do not fear death, although I worry about it. But I know that in my public and business activities I have made a difference. So I

44   http://www.quotationspage.com/quote/2471.html

say to you, my dear children, strive to make a difference. And I ask you to give me the greatest gift you can by embracing your mother if this disease takes me before I am ready—by embracing life, embracing love, and embracing each other. And in that embrace, be the best person, son, brother, sister, husband, mother, and father you can be.

As you live your lives, make the most of them. Live out your dreams.

*One Moment in Time*[45]

Give me one moment in time
When I'm more than I thought I could be
—Whitney Houston

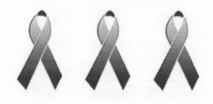

45   http://www.lyrics007.com/Whitney%20Houston%20Lyrics/One%20Moment%2
     0In%20Time%20Lyrics.html

# CHAPTER 10

# A FINAL WORD

*A Place in the Sun*[46]

And before my life is done
Got to find me a place in the sun.
—Stevie Wonder

Indeed we are all trying to find our place in the sun. It is probably more urgent for people like me who have more of a clock on our lives, but all of us think about it to one degree or another.

This book is a work of my life in progress. There was a beginning fifty-four years ago when I was born, and thankfully I have survived a major health challenge. And now I must find my new place in the sun.

In the time between when I "finished" this book and was preparing it for publication, the flow of difficulties did not end. I suffered more episodes of blackouts, one of which resulted in a fractured leg. I spent two more times in the hospital for respiratory problems, and

---

46  http://www.lyrics007.com/Stevie%20Wonder%20Lyrics/A%20Place%20In%20T
he%20Sun%20Lyrics.html

finally I had a problem that is similar to something called hydroceph-alus and is called a hygromas. Common in very young children and the elderly, this condition means that the lining around my brain no longer naturally absorbs my spinal fluid. As a result, the fluid collects around my brain, creating pressure and massive headaches. I had surgery to drain the fluid once in early 2007 and have had several more limited procedures that also drained the fluid from around my brain. To give you a feel for the limited procedure, the doctor took a large needle, inserted it into my skull (I had no anesthesia or numb-ing medicine), and withdrew the fluid. It is quite painful, to say the least!! My doctors are now trying to determine a long-term solution to the problem because it will never get better.

Unfortunately, the only way to address the problem is to install a permanent drain that will divert the fluid from my brain to my abdomen, but that presents a significant infection risk that could be fatal to someone like me that is immunocompromised. Therefore, we continue to explore options. Meanwhile, the massive headaches and weekly painful drainages continue.

These are the risks and complications that someone like me faces long term, but they are just that—risks, things that I have to deal with and live with.

I am realistic about my chances for long-term survival and aware that I have been cheating death over the last few years. Less than 20 percent of those with my disease survive for more than five years past the date of their transplant. And many I knew were not among them.

None of you reading this book know whether today is your last day or last week or last year for that matter. Many of you will be for-tunate enough to live your life without the threat of major illness.

I know that my complications may continue. In fact, I have come to know that they will. It seems as though when I conquer one battle, another complication raises its ugly head. That just seems to be what has been prescribed for me, at least for now. I have not spent my last days in the hospital. I still must take naps daily and do not know what tomorrow will bring. I continue to take about forty medications daily, including pills, patches, and injections. Some days are better than others. Some days I feel well; some days I don't feel so well. But that is just the way it is.

I have also just learned that my heart function has continued to decline to the point that my last echocardiogram measured the function at 27 percent and that I am in constant congestive heart failure with a pulse rate running constantly at over 120 beats per minute. That is also a very serious condition that must be contained.

For those of us who either have walked or are now walking this road, it is a hard and painful one indeed—not only for yourselves but for your families, friends, and loved ones. Perhaps the most difficult thing I have ever had to do was to tell my children, friends, and loved ones that I had a life-threatening disease—not knowing whether we all would have the time together that we had once envisioned.

This road has caused pain for me, agony for my family, and upset for my friends, and it seems to never end. In fact, it is said that more people die from the side effects and aftereffects of leukemia than from the disease itself. For me, the complications and post-treatment hospitalizations have been a struggle, and I now know that I will deal with them for the rest of my life.

But you will grow from this experience as well. Pamela and I loved each other from the beginning and have learned how to love each other more as the years passed. More than that we learned how to live with adversity and uncertainty. We have learned how to face the unknown and how to face the prospect of death.

But we all need to move on as best we can. We must persevere. We are given the gift of life, and it is our duty to live it to the best of our ability—to make things better because we lived on Earth. We would cheat ourselves and shortchange our families and friends if we did not give life all that we have to offer.

In the beginning, I told you not to dwell on the on negatives or the "why" of getting cancer. Instead you will get through your ordeal by focusing on what you will do with the rest of your life. Your life after cancer will be different in many ways, but you will find that your creativity and resiliency can carry you through even the most difficult times.

In other words, you should decide how you will respond when cancer calls.

I clearly am not the same man today that I was the day before I was diagnosed with leukemia. Facing mortality brings home the need to do all of those things that people say they should do: spend more time with friends and family; live a more balanced life; stop and smell the roses. These are clichés until they become real, which for me they are now.

Facing mortality in the short term also brings up many questions. It tests your core beliefs about life and what follows life on Earth. Is there a heaven? Have I earned entry? Have I done enough good on this Earth to be judged by my peers, friends, colleagues, and loved ones as someone who made the most out of life? Will I be missed? Will I leave a legacy for the future? Will there be concrete evidence that I walked this way? It is just natural to have these questions.

I said earlier that the day you are diagnosed will change your life forever. Take it from me, you simply will need to change the way you live your life.

My son has a great expression for it; he tells me to keep an even keel. I imagine myself like a ship on the sea. As long as I stay righted, I will sail right along. But if I lose my even keel, I risk falling over and sinking.

One of the most difficult things for me was to put my work life behind me. I was always motivated by work and by the benefits it brought to my family. I had a wonderful job that was visible, exciting, and fun. What's more is that it allowed me to continue the work I began when I was eighteen and on the city council—working in my community to make a difference. But for now my body cannot cash the checks that my mind is writing. I don't have the stamina anymore to do that work on a full-time basis, so I had to leave that behind.

But I am not through trying to make a difference. However, now my focus is on people whom cancer has called. I want to use my remaining time working to spread the word about bone marrow transplants and even more importantly about how we all can do better for patients by focusing on caregivers, wellness, and patient survivorship. To that end, perhaps the highest priority I have will be to focus on establishing a Silicon Valley affiliate of The Wellness Community, the country's gold standard for dealing with the psychosocial needs of cancer patients, caregivers, families and loved ones. The medical community does a great job dealing with the medical needs of patients; however the psychosocial and support needs are not as well met and not focused. Pamela and I were fortunate that there was a Wellness Community facility available to us in Los Angeles, however there is not one in Silicon Valley. We are committed to opening one there in the not too distant future.

Above all, we will improve the chances for people with cancer most by eliminating the environmental factors and personal habits that increase ones risk of getting cancer in the first place. Although we do not know what causes cancer in all cases, we know that there are certain things that do.

We must work to clean our air so that people do not inhale deadly pollutants. We must do everything in our power to convince people to stop smoking. Promoting healthy eating will help as well. More work needs to be done to eliminate chemicals that we know produce predispositions to cancer. Government and private industry must spend whatever it takes to find cures. The amount of money we are spending in finding cures is miniscule in comparison to what we spend treating the diseases after people get it, much less the money government wastes every day without even thinking about it.

Promoting early detection is a part of my mission as well. I was told that if my leukemia had gone undetected for six months to a year, I would have had a grim outcome due to the acute nature of my disease. I know that colonoscopies are embarrassing and uncomfortable. But don't avoid them when you reach fifty. It could save your life. Don't neglect the annual physical exam. Although my leukemia was not discovered by my annual physical, the blood tests given during the annual exam often uncover abnormal blood counts that can unveil blood cancers.

None of us know when our lives will end or whether the end will be by accident or illness. It is therefore essential that you live your life every day as though it will be your last.

Life is not what we always hope it will be; nor can it be planned the way we want to plan it. Yesterday is gone and tomorrow is uncertain, so we must live for today

I am not one who believes that you should let go of the past, but I do believe that you should not dwell on it. We all have things about the past we would change—mistakes we made or regrets from things that happened. It is good therapy to document them and leave them behind. By documenting them, you can resolve to right the wrongs and undo what you can as priorities in your return to wellness.

But if we walk with courage, faith, and determination—one step at a time—we can make the best of the future that we are capable of.

I cannot say that the journey has been easy to this point. I cannot say that there were not days of despair, nights of anger, and periods of loneliness. There were days when I regretted my decision to proceed with treatment rather than take my chances and live out my life to the best quality I could achieve—and without being a burden on so many people. Nor can I say that I did not pray for relief from the suffering for me and my loved ones. But whenever I reached those depths, thoughts of my wife, children, and all of those who supported me throughout my ordeal gave me the courage and determination to fight on.

I said earlier that cancer knows no boundaries. I don't know why I got leukemia, but there must be a reason. I guess I have concluded that, since I can't explain why empirically, there must be a higher reason that I was given this challenge. Perhaps it is because I have now been enlisted as a soldier in the fight against cancer or as a megaphone to expand transplant donors. Whatever the reason, I know that a portion of the rest of my life will be dedicated to making life better for cancer patients, their families, friends, and loved ones.

Beginning with this book, I am committing myself to being an evangelist to help people deal with the life-changing experiences Pamela, Gerald, Jennifer, and I have dealt with. One way I hope to do this is as a member of the board of directors of the National Marrow Donor Program, a position I was elected to at the beginning of 2007.

This is my story—to this point. I don't know whether I will beat cancer or whether it will beat me. I am grateful that I have survived long enough to write this book and share with you my experiences and my observations. I still have struggles ahead—ones that I cannot even see or define today. But I will do all I can to make the best of every day that is given to me.

Remember, having cancer does not mean that you are entering the last phase of your life. You are entering a new phase, and the only thing that matters is what you choose to do with it.

How will you respond when cancer calls?

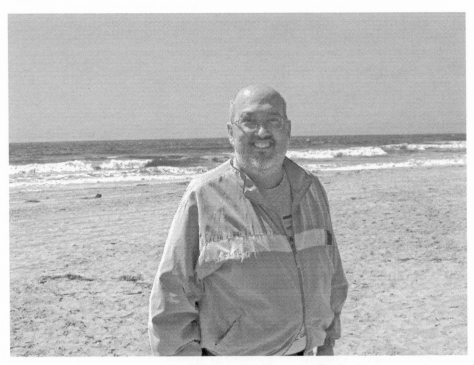

One of my favorite beach locations, Pajaro Dunes, California.

# APPENDIX A
# WHAT IS CANCER?

Cancer has been with us for at least three thousand five hundred years. But before getting into the history of the progress of cancer, let's talk about what cancer is.

Cancer simply starts when cells in one part of the body abnormally grow out of control. Unlike normal cells that have a specific purpose and grow, divide, and die, cancer cells grow out of control, turn into tumors (or do other damage), and create havoc in the body that damage tissue and form new abnormal cells. These cells then travel to other parts of the body where they begin to grow and replace normal tissue. This process, called metastasis, occurs as the cancer cells get into the bloodstream or lymph vessels.

Cancer is a very difficult disease to combat. It seems to invade all parts of the body. The death rate from cancer has been declining since 1991, and in 2003, the actual number of deaths declined for the first time in seventy years.[47]

Those with cancer need all of the hope, medicine, and healing they can avail themselves of. And they need the spiritual guidance

---

47  American Cancer Society. *Cancer Facts and Figures 2006.* Atlanta: American Cancer Society: 2006.

to get them through. The words of the following Hebrew prayer come to mind:

*Mi Sheberach*

*Mi sheberach avoteinu, m'kor*
*habraacha l'imoteinu*

(May the source of strength who
Blessed the ones before us
Help us find the courage to
Make our lives a blessing
And let us say, Amen)

*Mi sheberach imotenu, m'kor*
*habracha l'avoteinu*

(Bless those in need of healing with)

*Refuah shelamayh*

(The renewal of the body
The renewal of the spirit
And let us say, Amen)

In my introduction to this book, I asked you what type of cancer you have. I did so, not to scare you or sensationalize the disease, but to make sure you understand that we all have cells within us that either are or can become cancer. It is estimated that 1.4 million people will get cancer in 2006, and nearly 560,000 people will die of cancer in 2006.[48]

The table in this appendix summarizes new cancer cases and cancer-related death estimates for 2006.

Cancer can arise in any organ of the body, and it strikes one of every two American men and one of every three American women at some point in their lives.[49]

Cancer is the second leading cause of death in the United States. Half of all men and one-third of all women in the United States will develop cancer during their lifetimes. Today, millions of people are living with cancer or have had cancer.

The risk of developing most types of cancer can be reduced by changes in a person's lifestyle—for example, by quitting smoking and eating a better diet. The sooner a cancer is found and treatment begins, the better are the chances that the patient will live for many years.

## Cancer's history

Some of the earliest evidence of cancer is found among fossilized bone tumors, human mummies in ancient Egypt, and ancient manuscripts. Bone remains of mummies have revealed growths suggestive of the bone cancer, osteosarcoma. In other cases, bony skull destruction as seen in cancer of the head and neck has been found.

The first descriptions of cancer were discovered in Egypt in 1600 B.C. The Edwin Smith Papyrus describes cases of tumors that were

---

48  Ibid
49  Ibid.

treated by cauterization. The writing says about the disease, "There is no treatment."[50]

The word *cancer* is attributed to Hippocrates who used the terms *carrions* and *carcinoma* to describe tumors. In Greek these words refer to a crab, most likely applied to the disease because the finger-like spreading projections from a cancer called to mind the shape of a crab.[51]

The Scottish surgeon John Hunter (1728–1793) suggested that some cancers might be cured by surgery and described how the surgeon might decide which cancers to operate on. If the tumor had not invaded nearby tissue and was "moveable," he said, "There is no impropriety in removing it."[52]

A century later, the development of anesthesia allowed surgery to flourish, and the classic cancer operations such as radical mastectomy were developed.

By the nineteenth century, Rudolf Virchow, often called the founder of cellular pathology, provided the scientific basis for the modern pathologic study of cancer. This method not only allowed a better understanding of the damage cancer had done to a patient but also laid the foundation for the development of cancer surgery. Body tissues removed by the surgeon could now be examined and a precise diagnosis made. In addition, the pathologist could tell the surgeon whether the operation had completely removed the tumor.[53]

---

50   http://www.cancer.org/docroot/CRI/content/CRI_2_6x_the_history_of_cancer_72.asp?sitearea=CRI

51   Ibid.

52   http://www.rare-cancer.org/history-of-cancer.html

53   http://medicineworld.org/cancer/history.html

# Theories of cancer's causes[54]

There have been many theories through the years about the causes of cancer. New theories are continuing to develop. Some of these include:

- Exposure to substances such as tobacco, hydrocarbons, asbestos, radon, nickel, vinyl chloride, radiation, the sun, benzene, arsenic, etc.

- Diet, alcohol, and stress have been identified as potential causes.

- Enduring a longstanding liver infection from hepatitis (can lead to liver cancer).

- Contraction of a variety of the herpes virus called the Epstein-Barr virus (causes infectious mononucleosis and can cause non-Hodgkin's lymphomas and nasopharyngeal cancer).

- Contraction of the HIV virus (associated with an increased risk of developing several cancers, especially Kaposi's sarcoma and non-Hodgkin's lymphoma).

- Contraction of the human papilloma viruses (HPVs) (linked to cancers of the cervix, throat, vulva, and penis).

---

54   http://www.medicinenet.com/cancer_causes/page2.htm

# How cancer starts[55,56]

Cancer is a word that refers to approximately fifty diseases that exhibit two characteristics in common: (1) an uncontrolled growth of cells and (2) the ability to invade and damage normal tissues either locally or at distant sites in the body. Cancer is caused by a series of mutations, or alterations, in genes that control cells' ability to grow and divide. Some mutations are inherited; others arise from environmental or other factors.

Every cancer therefore starts with a single cell that has been released from the restraints placed on all normal cells. Because the changes that have taken place within the cancer cell have been directed by the cell's DNA, they are passed on to each of the cells arising from the original cancer cell. Eventually, a family of abnormal cells is formed. Except in the case of leukemia, these cells form a mass, or tumor. In the case of leukemia, these cells remain in the blood or marrow.

The cells of the tumor then push outward from their boundaries, invading surrounding normal tissues. Small clumps of cells may then dislodge from the tumor and migrate to distant sites, often by invading the circulatory system of the blood or lymph glands. After traveling to a new organ, the cancer cells invade the surrounding tissues. There they continue to multiply, forming secondary tumors in a process called metastasis.

These cells are already within our bodies—they become cancers when our systems are no longer able to prevent them from uncontrollably dividing and thus doing damage to tissues, bones,

---

55   http://cancerguide.org/basic.html
56   http://www.cancer.gov/cancertopics/wyntk/overview/page3

or organs. As a result, the cells do not die off in an orderly manner and form tumors. Tumors that grow uncontrollably are called malignant tumors. This occurs when our DNA can no longer send the appropriate signals to the cells and thus alter the normal growth of the cells. DNA can be altered by many factors—chief among them are exposures to radiation, chemicals, other substances such as those from smoking, using drugs, or other activities. Or it could occur because there are fundamental flaws in a person's DNA, as opposed to it having been caused by things we may do to ourselves. In any case, the DNA breaks or mutates, and when it recombines, the cell containing it can no longer produce the normal protein whose function is to suppress cancer.

Carcinomas, the most common type of cancer, originate in tissues that cover a surface or line a cavity of the body. Sarcomas begin in tissue that connect, support, or surround other tissues and organs. Lymphomas are cancers of the lymph system, the circulatory system that bathes and cleanses the body's cells. Leukemias involve blood-forming tissues and blood cells. As their names indicate, brain tumors are cancers that begin in the brain, and skin cancers, including dangerous melanomas, originate in the skin. Cancers are considered metatastic if they spread via the blood or lymphatic system to other parts of the body to form secondary tumors.

## Treatment[57]

Generally, the treatment for cancer includes some or all of the following treatments:

---

57   http://www.cancer.gov/cancertopics/treatment

- <u>Surgery</u> is one of the most longstanding treatments for cancer. For many types of cancer it offers the greatest chance of cure, especially when the cancer is limited to a specific organ and has not metastasized. It also has an important role in diagnosing and staging (finding the extent) of cancer. Advances in surgical techniques have allowed surgeons to successfully operate on a growing number of patients. Today, more limited (less invasive) operations are often done to remove tumors while preserving as much normal function as possible.

- <u>Chemotherapy</u> involves the use of toxic drugs to kill cancer cells. Unfortunately, chemotherapy drugs also kill good cells at the same time.

- <u>Radiation treatments</u> use radioactive therapies, which are aimed at specific tumors in an attempt to destroy the tumors. Radiation can also be administered to segments of or to the entire body, also known as total body irradiation (TBI). Radiation therapy attacks reproducing cancer cells, but it can also affect the reproduction of cells of normal tissues. The damage to normal cells is what causes side effects. Each time radiation therapy is given, it involves a balance between destroying the cancer cells and sparing the normal cells.

- <u>Bone marrow/stem cell transplants</u> are a treatment in which a patient's immune system is replaced by that of a donor.

- <u>Alternative therapies</u> use nutrition, vitamins, exercise, and other non-medical treatments.

- <u>Newly emerging medical advances</u> include gene therapy, photodynamic therapy, immunotherapy, monoclonal antibodies, cancer vaccines, and other new advances.

Each type of cancer responds differently to different treatments and not all options are applicable to every cancer. Your medical specialist is the best one to counsel patients on the best available treatment.

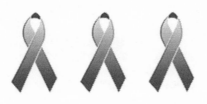

# Estimated New Cancer Cases and Deaths in US—2006

|  | New Cases | | | Deaths | | |
|---|---|---|---|---|---|---|
|  | Both sexes | Male | Female | Both sexes | Male | Female |
| All cancers | 1,399,790 | 720,280 | 679,510 | 545,830 | 291,270 | 273,560 |
| Oral | 30,990 | 20,180 | 10,810 | 7,430 | 5,050 | 2,380 |
| Digestive system | 263,060 | 137,630 | 125,430 | 136,180 | 75,210 | 60,970 |
| Respiratory system | 186,370 | 101,900 | 84,470 | 167,050 | 93,820 | 73,230 |
| Bones/joints | 2,760 | 1,500 | 1,260 | 1,260 | 730 | 530 |
| Soft tissues | 9,530 | 5,720 | 3,810 | 3,500 | 1,830 | 1,670 |
| Skin | 68,780 | 38,360 | 30,420 | 10,710 | 6,990 | 3,720 |
| Breast | 214,640 | 1,720 | 212,920 | 41,430 | 460 | 40,970 |
| Reproductive | 321,490 | 244,240 | 77,250 | 56,060 | 28,000 | 28,060 |
| Urinary | 102,740 | 70,940 | 31,800 | 26,670 | 17,530 | 9,140 |
| Eye | 2,360 | 1,230 | 1,130 | 230 | 110 | 120 |
| Brain | 18,820 | 10,730 | 8,090 | 12,820 | 7,260 | 5,560 |
| Endocrine | 32,260 | 8,690 | 23,570 | 2,290 | 1,020 | 1,270 |
| Lymphoma | 66,670 | 34,870 | 31,800 | 20,330 | 10,770 | 9,560 |
| Multiple Myeloma | 16,570 | 9,250 | 7.320 | 11,310 | 5,680 | 5,630 |
| Leukemia | 35,070 | 20,000 | 15,070 | 22,280 | 12,470 | 9,810 |
| Other | 27,680 | 13,320 | 14,360 | 45,280 | 24,340 | 20,94 |

Source: American Cancer Society. *Cancer Facts and Figures 2006.* Atlanta: American Cancer
    Society: 2006

# APPENDIX B
## ABOUT LEUKEMIA

I did not know very much about leukemia before I began this journey. My impression was that it was a disease that primarily impacted young people. I was wrong. Adults are at more risk of this disease than are children.

Leukemia is a malignant cancer of the bone marrow and blood. It occurs due to the uncontrolled growth and multiplication of blood cells, and comes in two classes: acute and chronic leukemias. Within each of these two classes, the leukemia is further classified as myelogenous or lymphocytic leukemias, based on the types of cells that are involved. Thus, the four principal types of leukemia are:

- Acute Lymphocytic Leukemia (ALL)
- Acute Myelogenous Leukemia (AML)
- Chronic Lymphocytic Leukemia (CLL)
- Chronic Myelogenous Leukemia (CML)

## Acute Lymphocytic Leukemia (ALL)[58]

Acute lymphocytic leukemia may also be referred to as acute lymphoid leukemia and acute lymphoblastic leukemia.

ALL begins with a change to a single cell in the bone marrow. Scientists are studying the exact genetic changes that cause a normal cell to become an ALL cell. In ALL, too many stem cells develop into a type of white blood cell called lymphocytes. The lymphocytes may also be called lymphoblasts or leukemic cells. There are three types of lymphocytes: B Lymphocytes that make antibodies to help fight infection, T Lymphocytes that help B lymphocytes make the antibodies that help fight infection, and natural killer cells that attack cancer cells and viruses.

In ALL, the lymphocytes are not able to fight infection very well. Also, as the number of lymphocytes increases in the blood and bone marrow, there is less room for healthy white blood cells, red blood cells, and platelets. As a result, people develop red blood cell, platelet, and white cell deficiencies.

In addition to the symptoms described below for AML, those with ALL may find that lymph nodes can become enlarged as the lymphoblasts accumulate in the lymphatic system, and they may experience headaches and vomiting as the cells accumulate in the brain or spinal cord.

The prognosis for recovery is impacted by the age of the patient, whether the cancer has spread to the brain or spinal cord, and whether the cancer has been treated before. Patients with ALL need to start chemotherapy right away. Allogeneic stem cell transplant is a treatment generally used for adult patients with ALL but is

---

58   http://www.leukemia-lymphoma.org/all_page?item_id=7049

not recommended for younger patients unless chemotherapy and radiation do not achieve a remission.

## Acute Myelogenous Leukemia[59]

Acute myelogenous leukemia (AML) can be referred to as: acute myelocytic leukemia, acute myeloblastic leukemia, acute granulocytic leukemia, or acute nonlymphocytic leukemia.

AML results from genetic damage to the DNA of cells. This cell damage results in the uncontrolled growth of cells that are called "leukemic blasts." Leukemia cells are unable to do their usual work and can build up in the bone marrow and blood so there is less room for healthy white blood cells, red blood cells, and platelets. When this happens, infection, anemia, or easy bleeding may occur. The leukemia cells can spread outside the blood to other parts of the body, including the central nervous system (brain and spinal cord), skin, and gums. AML is not contagious nor is it inherited.

Most people with AML do not have significant symptoms that cause them to seek medical assistance. However, it is an acute medical condition that requires immediate mediate medical attention. Generally, people with AML feel a loss of energy due to anemia. They tire more easily and may feel short of breath. They may bleed or bruise easily with only minor bumps. They may also develop pin-head-sized spots under the skin, called petechiae, or have prolonged bleeding from minor cuts. Fevers, swollen gums, bone pain, and minor infections are other possible signs of AML.

AML is generally detected in one of the following ways:

59   http://www.leukemia-lymphoma.org/all_page?item_id=8459

- <u>Physical exam</u> to check general signs of health, including checking for signs of disease, such as lumps or anything else that seems unusual. A history of the patient's health habits and past illnesses and treatments could also be useful in detecting AML. A complete blood count, via a procedure in which a sample of blood is drawn and checked for the numbers of red cells, white cells, platelets, and the amount of hemoglobin in the red blood cells, will be determined.

- <u>Blood chemistry studies,</u> in which a blood sample is checked to measure the amounts of certain substances released into the blood by organs and tissues in the body. An unusual (higher or lower than normal) amount of a substance can be a sign of disease in the organ or tissue that produces it.

- <u>Peripheral blood smear</u>, in which a sample of blood is checked for the presence of blast cells, number and kinds of white blood cells, the number of platelets, and changes in the shape of blood cells.

- <u>Bone marrow aspiration and biopsy</u>, a procedure in which a small piece of bone and bone marrow are extracted by inserting a needle into the hip bone or breastbone.

- <u>Cytogenesis analysis,</u> a test in which the cells in a sample of blood or bone marrow are viewed under a microscope to look for certain changes in the chromosomes.

- <u>Immunophenotyping</u> is a process used to identify cells, based on the types of antigens or markers on the surface of the cell. This process is used to diagnose the subtype of AML by comparing the cancer cells to normal cells of the immune system.

Additional techniques used in the diagnostic process include γ-rays, CT scan, MRI scan, spinal tap, and ultrasound. These techniques, and those I described above, are effective for diagnosing leukemias, regardless of classification.

The prognosis (chance of recovery) and treatment for patients with AML depend upon the age of the patient, the subtype of AML, whether the patient received chemotherapy in the past to treat a different cancer, whether there is a history of a blood disorder, whether the cancer has spread to the central nervous system, and whether the cancer has been treated before or recurred.

It is important that acute leukemia be treated right away.

## Chronic Lymphocytic Leukemia (CLL)[60]

Chronic Lymphocytic Leukemia (CLL) results from an acquired injury to the DNA of a single cell, a lymphocyte, in the bone marrow that is not present at birth. Scientists do not yet understand what produces this change in the DNA of CLL patients.

The change in the cell's DNA results in the uncontrolled growth of CLL cells in the marrow, leading to an increased concentration in the blood. The lymphocytes in CLL, B lymphocytes, T lymphocytes, and natural killer cells) are not able to fight infection very well. Also, as the amount of lymphocytes increases in the blood and bone marrow, there is less room for healthy white blood cells, red blood cells, and platelets. This may result in infection, anemia, and easy bleeding. The CLL cells that accumulate in the marrow do not impede normal blood cell production to the extent that is

60   http://www.leukemia-lymphoma.org/all_page?item_id=7059

the case in other leukemias. This important distinction from acute leukemia accounts for the less severe early course of the disease.

Chronic lymphocytic leukemia does not result from exposure to high-dose radiation or benzene exposures, as is the case with the other three major types of leukemia. CLL is very uncommon in individuals under forty-five years of age. At the time of diagnosis, about 95 percent of patients are over age fifty, and the incidence of the disease increases dramatically thereafter.

Early in the disease, chronic lymphocytic leukemia may have little effect on an individual. The symptoms of CLL usually develop gradually and are similar to other leukemias. In addition, patients may experience infections of the skin, lungs, kidneys, or other organs.

Many CLL patients say they learned they had CLL after a routine check-up when an enlarged lymph node or an enlarged spleen is found, or when a routine blood test shows a higher than normal number of lymphocytes.

The prognosis for recovery is impacted by the stage of the disease, Red blood cell, white blood cell, and platelet blood counts, whether there are symptoms, such as fever, chills, or weight loss, whether the liver, spleen, or lymph nodes are larger than normal, and the patient's general health.

## Chronic Myelogenous Leukemia (CML)[61]

Chronic myelogenous leukemia may be called by several names, including chronic granulocytic, chronic myelocytic, or chronic myeloid leukemia.

---

61   http://www.leukemia-lymphoma.org/all_page?item_id=8501

CML results from an acquired injury to the DNA of a stem cell in the marrow. This injury is not present at birth. Scientists do not yet understand what produces this change in the DNA in patients with CML.

As a result of this DNA change, the individual experiences an uncontrolled growth of white blood cells. Unlike AML, chronic myelogenous leukemia permits the development of normally-functioning white blood cells. This important distinction from acute leukemia accounts for the less severe early course of the disease.

Most cases of chronic myelogenous leukemia occur in adults. Only 2.6 percent of leukemias in children ages zero to nineteen are CML.

Chronic myelogenous leukemia is unlike other leukemias due to the presence of a genetic abnormality in blood cells, called the Philadelphia chromosome. The changes that result in this chromosome "causing" chronic myelogenous leukemia have been studied intensively. The chromosome in CML patients is shorter in length than that of the same chromosome in normal cells. They named this shortened chromosome the Philadelphia chromosome, because the observation was made at the University of Pennsylvania School of Medicine in that city. The defect in the Philadelphia chromosome is *not* passed from parent to child.

In addition, chromosome numbers 9 and 22 are generally abnormal.

The cause of the chromosomal abnormality in virtually all CML patients is not known. In a small proportion of patients, the cause of the breakage is exposure to very high doses of radiation. This effect has been most carefully studied in the Japanese survivors of the atomic bomb, whose leukemia risk was significantly increased. A slight increase in risk also occurs in some individuals treated with high dose radiotherapy for other cancers, such as lymphoma. Exposures to diagnostic dental or medical X-rays have not been associated with a heightened risk of chronic myelogenous leukemia.

In addition to many of the same symptoms of other leukemias, patients also feel discomfort on the left side of the abdomen from an enlarged spleen is a frequent complaint. Patients may experience excessive sweating, weight loss and inability to tolerate warm temperatures. The disease is generally discovered during the course of a "routine" medical examination when blood tests reveal the high level of white cells.

Most of the tests used to detect other leukemias are also used to diagnose CML.

The prognosis for patients with CML generally depend upon the patient's age, the phase of CML, the amount of blasts in the blood or bone marrow, the size of the spleen at diagnosis, and the patient's general health.

Acute leukemias are rapidly progressing diseases, whereas chronic leukemias progresses much more slowly. As a result, acute leukemias require urgent attention and medical care and are more serious. Chronic leukemia can be observed and treated over a longer period of time.

An estimated 44,240 new cases of leukemia are expected to be diagnosed in the United States in 2007. Acute leukemias were expected to account for nearly seven percent more of the cases than chronic leukemias. Most cases of acute leukemia occur in older adults; more than half of all cases occur after age sixty-seven. Leukemia strikes ten times as many adults as children. Approximately 33 percent of cancers in children ages zero to fourteen years are leukemia, and leukemia is the most common form of death from cancer for young people. The most common form of leukemia among children under nineteen years of age is ALL.

The most common type of leukemia among adults is AML, with an estimated 15,340 in 2007, and CLL, with some 13,410 new cases. CML is estimated to affect about 4,570 persons, and ALL will account for about 3,970 cases in 2005. Other unclassified forms of leukemia account for the 5,200 cases.

Men tend to be at slightly higher risks for leukemia than are women. In 2005, males were expected to account for more than 56 percent of the cases of leukemia.[62]

Leukemia is one of the top fifteen most frequently occurring cancers in minority groups. Leukemia incidence is highest among whites and lowest among American Indians/Alaskan natives. Leukemia rates are substantially higher for white children than for black children.

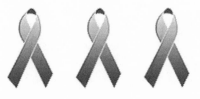

# Appendix C
# Resources

There are thousands of not-for-profit organizations, foundations, and government agencies throughout the country doing great work in cancer. While it is not possible to list all of them, I have included below contact information on what I consider to be some of the major organizations that can be of help to you in investigating cancer and related subjects. This information was current as of the date of publication.

Additionally, the information revolution has drowned us in more information and material that we could ever consume. The Internet offers an excellent portal to do research, yet it can be overwhelming as well. Searches for cancer can yield links to so many Web sites that it is hard to know where to begin.

As a part of my ongoing work, I have developed a Web site that expands on these lists and provides a comprehensive listing of Web sites classified into useful categories. It will be constantly updated and I hope you will find it useful:

http://www.CancerWebLinks.com

# Cancer—General

American Association for Cancer Research
615 Chestnut Street, 17th Floor
Philadelphia, PA 19106-4404
Phone: 215-440-9300; Fax: 215-440-9372
http://www.aacr.org

American Cancer Society
1599 Clifton Road, NE
Atlanta, GA 30329-4251
Phone: 800-ACS-2345 (800-227-2345)
http://www.cancer.org

American Hospice Foundation
2120 L Street, NW, Suite 200
Washington, DC 20037-1547
Phone: 202-223-0204; Fax: 202-223-0208
http://www.americanhospice.org/

American Institute for Cancer Research
1759 R. Street, NW
Washington, DC 20009-2552
Phone: 800-843-8114; Fax: 202-328-7226
http://www.aicr.org

American Pain Foundation
201 N. Charles Street, Suite 710
Baltimore, MD 21201-4111

Phone: 888-615-PAIN (7246)
http://www.painfoundation.org

Association of Cancer Online Resources (ACOR.ORG)
173 Duane Street, Suite 3A
New York, NY 10013-3334
Phone: 212-226-5525
http://www.acor.org/

Association of Community Cancer Centers
11600 Nebel Street Suite 201
Rockville, MD 20852-2557
Phone: 301-984-9496; Fax: 301-770-1949
http://www.accc-cancer.org

Cancer Hope Network
Two North Road, Suite A
Chester, NJ 07930-2308
Phone: 877-HOPENET (467-3638); Fax: 908-879-6518
http://www.cancerhopenetwork.org

Cancer Trials Support Unit (CTSU)
1441 West Montgomery Avenue
Rockville, MD 20850-2062
Phone: 888-823-5923; Fax: 888-691-8039
http://www.ctsu.org/

Cancer.com
Ortho Biotech Products, L.P.

P.O. Box 6914
Bridgewater, NJ 08807-0914
Phone: 800-325-7504
http://www.cancer.com/

CancerCare, Inc.
275 7th Avenue, Floor 22
New York, NY 10001-6754
Phone: 800-813-HOPE (4673); Fax: 212-712-8495
http://www.cancercare.org

Coalition of National Cancer Cooperative Groups, Inc.
1818 Market Street, Suite 1100
Philadelphia, PA 19103-3611
Phone: 877-520-4457; Fax: 215-789-3655
http://www.cancertrialshelp.org

Gilda's Club Worldwide
322 Eighth Avenue, Suite 1402
New York, NY 10001-6773
Phone: 888-GILDA-4-U; Fax: 917-305-0549
http://www.gildasclub.org

Lance Armstrong Foundation/LIVESTRONG
P.O. Box 161150
Austin, TX 78716-1150
Phone: 512-236-8820; Fax: 512-236-8482
www.livestrong.org

National Cancer Institute
6116 Executive Boulevard
Room 3036 A
Bethesda, MD 20892-8322
www.cancer.gov

National Coalition for Cancer Survivorship
1010 Wayne Avenue, Suite 770
Silver Spring, MD 20910-5600
Phone: 877-622-7937; Fax: 301-565-9670
http://www.canceradvocacy.org

National Comprehensive Cancer Network (NCCN)
500 Old York Road, Suite 250
Jenkintown, PA 19046-2870
Phone: 888-909-6226; Fax: 215-728-3877
http://nccn.org

National Family Caregivers Association (NFCA)
10400 Connecticut Avenue, Suite 500
Kensington, MD 20895-3944
Phone: 800-896-3650; Fax: 301-942-2302
http://www.nfcacares.org/

National Hospice and Palliative Care Organization (NHPCO)
1700 Diagonal Road, Suite 625
Alexandria, VA 22314-2844
Phone: 800-658-8898; 703-837-1500

Fax: 703-837-1233
http://www.nhpco.org

OncoLink
Abramson Cancer Center of the University of Pennsylvania
3400 Spruce Street-2 Donner
Philadelphia, PA 19104-4283
Fax: 215-349-5445
http://www.oncolink.org

Patient Advocate Foundation
700 Thimble Shoals Blvd. Suite 200
Newport News, VA 23606-4532
Phone: 800-532-5274; Fax: 757-873-8999
http://www.patientadvocate.org/

The Mautner Project for Lesbians with Cancer
1707 L Street, Suite 230
Washington DC 20036-4222
Phone: 202-332-5536; Fax: 202-332-0662
http://www.mautnerproject.org

The Wellness Community
919 18th Street, NW
Suite 54
Washington, DC 20006-5503
Phone: 888-793-WELL; Fax: 202-659-9301
http://www.thewellnesscommunity.org

# Brain Cancer

American Brain Tumor Association (ABTA)
2720 River Road, Suite 146
Des Plaines, IL 60018-4106
Phone: 800-886-2282
Phone: 847-827-9910; Fax: 847-827-9918
http://www.abta.org/

National Brain Tumor Foundation (NBTF)
22 Battery Street, Suite 612
San Francisco, CA 94111-5520
Phone: 800-934-CURE (2873); Fax: 415-834-9980
http://www.braintumor.org

The Brain Tumor Foundation
1350 Avenue of the Americas, Suite 1200
New York, NY 10019-4702
Phone: 212-265-2401; Fax: 212-489-0203
http://www.braintumorfoundation.org

The Brain Tumor Society
124 Watertown Street, Suite 3-H
Watertown, MA 02472-2500
Phone: 800-770-TBTS; Fax: 617-924-9998
http://www.tbts.org

The Childhood Brain Tumor Foundation
20312 Watkins Meadow Drive

Germantown, MD 20876-4259
Phone: 301-515-2900; 877-217-4166
http://www.childhoodbraintumor.org

## Breast Cancer

FORCE: Facing Our Risk of Cancer Empowered
16057 Tampa Palms Blvd. W
PMB #373
Tampa, FL 33647-2001
Phone: 954-255-8732; Fax: 954-827-2200
http://www.facingourrisk.org

SHARE: Self-help for Women with Breast/Ovarian Cancer
1501 Broadway, Suite 704A
New York, NY 10036-5505
Phone: 866-891-2392
Phone: 212-719-0364; Fax: 212-869-3431
http://www.sharecancersupport.org

The National Breast Cancer Coalition (NBCC)
1101 17th Street, NW—Suite 1300
Washington, DC 20036-4710
Phone: 800-622-2838; Fax: 202-265-6854
http://www.natlbcc.org

The Susan G. Komen Breast Cancer Foundation, Inc.
5005 LBJ Freeway Suite 250
Dallas, TX 75244

Phone: (800-462-9273; Fax: 972-855-4300
http://www.komen.org/

Y-ME National Breast Cancer Organization, Inc.
212 West Van Buren Street, Suite 1000
Chicago, IL 60607-3903
Phone: Hotline, English: 800-221-2141
Hotline, Spanish: 800-986-9505
Fax: (312) 294-8597
http://www.y-me.org

## Cancer Centers—NCI-designated

NCI List of Comprehensive Cancer Centers
http://cancercenters.cancer.gov

## Children's Issues

Children's Brain Tumor Foundation
274 Madison Avenue, Suite 1004
New York, NY 10016-0701
Phone: 212-448-9494
http://www.cbtf.org

Make-A-Wish Foundation
3550 N. Central Avenue, Suite 300
Phoenix, AZ 85012-2127
Phone: 800-722-9474; Fax: 602-279-0855
http://www.wish.org

CureSearch: National Childhood Cancer Foundation
Children's Oncology Group
Research Operations Center
440 E. Huntington Drive-Suite 400
Arcadia, CA 91006-3776
Phone: 800-458-6223 (US and Canada Only)
Phone: 626-447-1674; Fax: 626-447-5295
http://www.curesearch.org

National Children's Cancer Society
1015 Locust, Suite 600
St. Louis, MO 63101-1322
Phone: 800-532-6459; Fax: 314-241-1996
http://www.nationalchildrenscancersociety.org

## Colorectal Cancer

Colon Cancer Alliance
5411 N. University Drive-Suite 202
Coral Springs, FL 33067-4637
Phone: 212-627-7451; Fax: 866-304-9075
http://www.ccalliance.org

Colorectal Cancer Network
P.O. Box 182
Kensington, MD 20895-0182
Phone: 301-879-1500; Fax: 267-821-7080
http://www.colorectal-cancer.net

# Eye Cancer

The Eye Cancer Network
Eye Care Foundation
115 E. 61st Street
New York, NY 10021-8183
Phone: 212-832-8170
http://www.eyecancer.com

# Gastrointestinal Cancer

GIST Support International
12 Bomaca Drive
Doylestown, PA 18901-2971
Phone: 215-340-9374; Fax: 215-340-1630
http://www.gistsupport.org/

# Head, Neck, and Oral Cancer

Support for People with Oral, Head, and Neck Cancer, Inc.
P.O. Box 53
Locust Valley, NY 11560-0053
Phone: 516-759-5333; Fax: 516-671-8794
http://www.spohnc.org

# Kidney Cancer

Kidney Cancer Association
1234 Sherman Avenue—Suite 203
Evanston, IL 60202-1375

Phone: 800-850-9132; Fax: 847-332-2978
http://www.kidneycancerassociation.org/

## Leukemia/Lymphoma

American Society for Blood and Marrow Transplantation
85 West Algonquin Road, Suite 550
Arlington Heights, IL 60005-4460
Phone: 847-427-0224; Fax: 847-427-9656
http://www.asbmt.org

BMT InfoNet
2310 Skokie Valley Road, Suite 104
Highland Park, IL 60035-1745
Phone: 888-597-7674
Phone: 847-433-3313; Fax: 847-433-4599
http://www.bmtinfonet.org/

Blood & Marrow Transplant Information Network
2900 Skokie Valley Road, Suite B
Highland Park, IL 60035-1000
Phone: 888-597-7674
Phone: 847-433-3313; Fax: 847-827-9918
http://www.bmtnews.org

Leukemia & Lymphoma Society
1311 Mamaroneck Avenue
White Plains, NY 10605-5221
Phone: 800-955-4572

Phone: 914-949-5213; Fax: 914-949-6691
http://www.leukemia.org

Lymphoma Research Foundation
8800 Venice Boulevard, Suite 207
Los Angeles, CA 90034-3256
Phone: 800-500-9976
Phone: 310-204-7040; Fax: 310-204-7043
http://www.lymphoma.org

National Marrow Donor Program
3001 Broadway Street, NE, Suite 500
Minneapolis, MN 55413-2197
Phone: 612-627-5800; 800-627-7692
http://www.marrow.org

National Bone Marrow Transplant Link
20411 West 12 Mile Road—Suite 108
Southfield, MI 48076-6404
Phone: 800-LINK-BMT (546-5268); 248-358-1886
http://www.nbmtlink.org/

## Liver Cancer

LiverTumor.org
967 North Shoreline Boulevard
Mountain View, CA 94043-1932
Phone: 877-306-3114; Fax: 650-390-8505
http://www.livertumor.org

# Lung Cancer

Alliance for Lung Cancer Advocacy, Support, & Education
500 West 8th Street, Suite 240
Vancouver, WA 98660-3086
Phone: 800-298-2436
Phone: 360-696-2436; Fax: 360-735-1305
http://www.alcase.org

American Lung Association
61 Broadway, 6th Floor
New York, NY 10006-2753
Phone: 800-LUNG-USA; Phone: 212-315-8700
http://www.lungusa.org

# Melanoma

Melanoma Research Foundation
170 Township Line Road, Bldg B
Hillsborough, NJ 08844-3867
Phone: 1-800-MRF-1290; Fax: 732-821-5955
http://www.melanoma.org

Skin Cancer Foundation
149 Madison Avenue, Suite 901
New York, NY 10016-8713
Phone: 800-SKIN-490
Phone: 212-725-5176; Fax: 212-725-5751
http://www.skincancer.org/

## Miscellaneous

National Institutes of Health Info. Database
http://www.medlineplus.gov

PDQ—Comprehensive Cancer Database of NCI
http://www.cancer.gov/cancerinfo/pdq

## Myeloma

International Myeloma Foundation
12650 Riverside Drive, Suite 206
North Hollywood, CA 91607-3466
Phone: 800-452-2873 (US and Canada only)
Phone: 818-487-7455; Fax: 818-487-7454
http://www.myeloma.org

## Ovarian Cancer

FORCE: Facing Our Risk of Cancer Empowered
16057 Tampa Palms Blvd.W
PMB #373
Tampa, FL 33647-2001
Phone: 954-255-8732; Fax: 954-827-2200
http://www.facingourrisk.org

Gilda Radner Familial Ovarian Cancer Registry
Roswell Park Cancer Institute
Elm and Carlton Streets
Buffalo, NY 14263-0001

Phone: 800-OVARIAN
http://www.ovariancancer.com

National Ovarian Cancer Coalition
500 NE Spanish River Boulevard, Suite 8
Boca Raton, FL 33431-4516
Phone: 888-OVARIAN
Phone: 561-393-0005; Fax: 561-393-7275
http://www.ovarian.org

## Pancreatic Cancer

Hirshberg Foundation for Pancreatic Cancer Research
375 Homewood Road
Los Angeles, CA 90049-2711
Phone: 310-472-6310; Fax: 310-471-1020
http://www.pancreatic.org

Pancreatic Cancer Action Network (PANCAN)
2141 Rosecrans Avenue, Suite 7000
El Segundo, CA 90245
Phone: 877-2-PANCAN; Fax: 310-725-0029
http://www.pancan.org

## Urologic Cancer

American Foundation for Urologic Disease
1128 N. Charles Street
Baltimore, MD 21201

Phone: 800-822-5277; Fax: 410-468-1808
http://www.afud.org

American Urological Association Foundation (AUA Foundation)
1000 Corporate Boulevard
Linthicum, MD 21090-2260
Phone: 866-746-4282; Fax: 410-689-3850

National Prostate Cancer Coalition
1158 15th Street NW
Washington, DC 20005-1706
Phone: 888-245-9455
Phone: 202-463-9455; Fax: 202-463-9456
http://www.4npcc.org

Us Too International, Inc.
Prostate Cancer Education and Support Network
5003 Fairview Avenue
Downers Grove, IL 60515-5286
Phone: 800-808-7866; Fax: 630-795-1602
http://www.ustoo.org

# Rare Cancers

National Organization for Rare Disorders (NORD)
55 Kenosia Avenue
PO Box 1968
Danbury, CT 06813-1968

Phone: 203-744-0100; Fax: 203-798-2291
http://www.rarediseases.org/

Rare Cancer Alliance
100 Tillotson St.
Canandaigua, NY 14424-2035
Phone: 520-625-5495; Fax: 909-609-3982
http://www.rare-cancer.org

## Thyroid Cancer

ThyCa: Thyroid Cancer Survivors' Association, Inc.
P.O. Box 1545
New York, NY 10159-1545
Phone: 877-588-7904; Fax: 503-905-9725
http://www.thyca.org

## Women's Issues

Gynecologic Cancer Foundation
230 W. Monroe, Suite 2528
Chicago, IL 60606-4902
Phone: 312-578-1439; Fax: 312-578-9769
http://www.wcn.org/gcf

# Live Help

If you would like to speak with someone by telephone about questions concerning cancer, U.S. residents may call the National Cancer Institute's (NCI's) Cancer Information Service toll-free at 1-800-4-CANCER (1-800-422-6237) Monday through Friday from 9:00 a.m. to 4:30 p.m, ET. Hearing impaired callers with TTY equipment may call 1-800-332-8615. The call is free, and a trained Cancer Information Specialist is available to answer your questions.

The Leukemia & Lymphoma Society has an information resource center. The center is open every business day to receive calls from 9 a.m. to 6 p.m. ET, at 1-800-955-4572. They also have specialists available live on the Internet as well at <u>www.lls.org</u>

## Publications

You will also find many publications available from organizations that are available free-of-charge. These publications discuss types of cancer, methods of cancer treatment, coping with cancer, and clinical trials. Some publications provide information on tests for cancer, cancer causes and prevention, cancer statistics, and NCI research activities. NCI materials on these and other topics may be ordered online or printed directly from the NCI Publications Locator. These materials can also be ordered by telephone from the Cancer Information Service toll-free at 1-800-4-CANCER (1-800-422-6237), TTY at 1-800-332-8615.

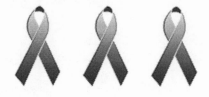

# APPENDIX D
# BEING NEUTROPENIC[63]

Neutropenia occurs in most cancer patients in the normal course of those treated with chemotherapy and or radiation when neutrophil granulocytes, which are a type of white blood cell, are too low. Since white cells are the body's primary source of defending against infections, the body has fewer defense mechanisms. As a result, patients must me placed on special diets and must also be very careful about cleanliness and take other special care.

Patients need to be extremely careful about the types of food they eat after the transplant. Food handling techniques are just as critical. Here is a summary of the foods and precautions:

- Cook meats until well done—there should be no remaining pink.

- Thaw meat, fish, or poultry in the refrigerator or microwave in a dish to catch drips. Use defrosted foods right away; do not refreeze.

---

63  City of Hope National Medical Center. "A Patient's Guide to Blood and Marrow Stem Cell Transplantation, 3rd Edition. 11/02.

- Never leave perishable food out of the refrigerator for over two hours. Egg dishes and cream- and mayonnaise-based foods should not be left unrefrigerated for more than one hour.

- Wash fruits and vegetables thoroughly under running water before peeling and cutting; cut away bruised areas.

- Wash tops of canned foods before opening. Wash can opener after each use with warm soapy water.

- During food preparation, do not taste the food with the same utensil used for stirring.

- Cook eggs until the whites are completely hard and the yokes begin to thicken. The yolk should no longer be runny, but they need not be hard.

Some items not allowed are:

- Dairy—Unpasteurized or raw milk, cheese, yogurt, and other milk products; cheeses from delicatessens; cheeses containing chili peppers or other uncooked vegetables; cheese with molds (i.e. blue, Stilton, Roquefort, and gorgonzola); sharp cheddar, brie, camembert, feta cheese, and farmers' cheese

- Vegetables, herbs and spices—Raw vegetables and salads; pepper; garnishes; uncooked herbs and spices

- Fruits and nuts—Dried fruits; raw fruit; un-pasteurized fruit and vegetable juices; raw nuts; roasted nuts in the shell; precut fresh fruits

- Bread, Grain, and Cereal Products—Raw grain products; Bakery breads, cakes, donuts, and muffins; potato/macaroni salad

- Meat and Meat Substitutes—Raw or undercooked meat, poultry, fish, game, and tofu; meats and cold cuts from a delicatessen; hard cured salami in natural wrap; cold smoked salmon and lox; pickled fish; sushi; raw oysters/clams

- Beverages—Well water; cold-brewed tea made with warm or cold water; sun tea; eggnog; fresh apple cider; homemade lemonade; spring water

- Deserts—Unrefrigerated cream-filled pastry products (not shelf-stable); cream- or custard-filled donuts; raw or unpasteurized honey; herbal and nontraditional (health food store) nutritional supplements, Chinese herbs; brewers yeast, if eaten uncooked

Home Sanitation is also important. More germs are transmitted through inadequate hand washing and lack of good home sanitation than any other method. To a person with a compromised immune system, these can be deadly. Some precautions that help:

- Wash hands with anti-bacterial soap and warm, running water before and after every step in food preparation.
- Wash hands before eating, using the rest room, touching pets, etc.
- Dry hands with paper towels and dispose of them.
- Wash hands after shaking hands with anyone.

- Use separate cutting boards for cooked and raw foods.

- Replace dishcloths and dish towels daily.

- Use liquid dish soap when and washing dishes and pans.

- Maintain refrigerator temperature between 34° F. 40° F.

- Maintain freezer temperature to below 5° F.

- Discard foods older than their "use by" expiration dates; discard all prepared foods after seventy-two hours (three days).

- Discard freezer-burned foods.

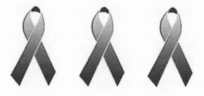

# APPENDIX E
# THE NATIONAL MARROW
# DONOR PROGRAM[64]

The National Marrow Donor Program (NMDP) is the critical link in the chain between patients who need a lifesaving transplant and donors interested in offering their stem cells, bone marrow, or cord blood. Those patients who have relatives that match them or for whom a self-donation or autologous transplant is an option do not rely on the NMDP. But for those who do not have those options, the NMDP is their lifesaver.

The (NMDP) helps people who need a lifesaving marrow or blood cell transplant. They connect patients, doctors, donors, and researchers to resources they need to help more people live longer, healthier lives.

Today, more than six million people have registered through the NMDP to be potential donors. However, that is no where near enough to meet the need. Many of these people may no longer qualify to be donors. They may no longer be within the age limits (up to sixty) to qualify. They may have since suffered an intervening

---

64   I am aware of the information contained in this appendix as a result of being a member of the Board of Directors of the National Marrow Donor Program. More information about the NMDP may be obtained at www.nmdp.org.

illness that disqualifies them. They may have changed their mind. Other life changes could have intervened to disqualify them. Some may have registered to match one specific person and may decline another; but it only takes one special person to match one special person. In the end, millions more are needed simply because our world and our cultures are becoming even more intermingled every day meaning that DNA combinations are becoming intermingled.

Today, with millions of potential donors and tens of thousands of cord blood units on the registry, the likelihood of finding an unrelated donor is increasing for patients from all racial and ethnic groups.

Unfortunately, some patients are unable to find a match because of the rarity of their tissue types. Because tissue types are inherited, their most likely match is with someone from the same racial or ethnic group. That is why a pressing need remains for more people who identify themselves as American Indian or Alaska Native, Asian, Black or African American, Hispanic or Latino, Native Hawaiian or Other Pacific Islander, or multiple-race to volunteer as donors or to donate umbilical cord blood.

Investment in Umbilical Cord Blood—Umbilical cord blood is playing an important and growing role in the treatment of leukemia and other life-threatening diseases. The NMDP's Center for Cord Blood coordinates a growing network of cord blood banks.

Donor Education and Recruitment—To connect more patients with donors, the NMDP works with families, communities, businesses and other groups to raise awareness and recruit committed individuals to join the registry. Recruitment efforts focus on increasing the diversity of tissue types and recruiting people who will stay committed and available to help any patient in need.

<u>Donor Advocacy</u>—Through its Donor Advocacy Program, the NMDP supports donors through every step of the donation process. To contact the Donor Advocacy Program, send e-mail to <u>advocate@nmdp.org</u> or call 1-800-526-7809 (toll-free in the United States). Outside the United States, call 1-612-627-5800.

Many patients who could be treated with a marrow or blood cell transplant face barriers and challenges. The National Marrow Donor Program is committed to removing these barriers and offers support to patients through its Office of Patient Advocacy (OPA).

Patients and physicians can contact the National Marrow Donor Program Office of Patient Advocacy at 1-888-999-6743 (toll-free in the United States). Outside of the United States, call 1-612-627-8140.

- Since it began operations in 1987, the National Marrow Donor Program has facilitated more than twenty-five thousand marrow or blood cell transplants for patients who do not have matching donors in their families.
- On average, the NMDP facilitates more than two hundred sixty transplants each month, with more than three thousand two hundred marrow and cord blood transplants in 2006.
- Patients diagnosed with leukemia, lymphomas or other blood cancers make up approximately 73 percent of transplants facilitated by the NMDP. The remaining patients undergo transplant to treat a variety of immune system and inherited disorders.

- Only 30 percent of patients in need of a marrow or blood cell transplant find a matched donor in their family. The other 70 percent may turn to the NMDP to search for an unrelated donor or cord blood unit.

- Lack of financial resources can delay donor searches or limit opportunities for post-transplant care. For patients who qualify for financial assistance, the NMDP offers The Marrow Foundation Patient Assistance Program. In 2006, more than one thousand requests for funds were approved and more than four million dollars were made available to patients in need.

- On average, twenty-five thousand new volunteers join the NMDP Registry each month, making over three hundred thousand new volunteers each year.

- The NMDP's Center for Cord Blood provides more than fifty thousand cord blood units from nineteen member blood banks.

- The NMDP maintains relationships with donor centers, transplant centers and other registries in thirty-five countries outside of the United States, and more than 40 percent of all transplants facilitated by the NMDP involve an international donor or recipient.

## Patients Served Since 1987, by Race and Ethnicity

| | |
|---|---|
| American Indian/Alaska Native | More than 100 |
| Asian | More than 680 |
| Black or African American | More than 1,000 |

| | |
|---|---|
| Native Hawaiian/Pacific Islander | More than 15 |
| White | More than 20,000 |
| Hispanic | More than 1,600 |
| **Total** | More than 23,400 |

## Diversity of the NMDP Registry—Adult Donors
## Adult Volunteers on the NMDP Registry by Race

| | |
|---|---|
| American Indian/Alaska Native | More than 75,000 |
| Asian | More than 415,000 |
| Black or African American | More than 480,000 |
| Native Hawaiian/Pacific Islander | More than 8,000 |
| White | More than 3 million |
| Multiple Race | More than 150,000 |
| Unknown* | More than 1.5 million |
| **Total** | More than 6 million |

## Adult Volunteers on the NMDP Registry by Ethnicity

| | |
|---|---|
| Hispanic or Latino | More than 580,000 |
| Non-Hispanic | More than 5.5 million |
| **Total** | More than 6 million |

Updated annually (last update February 2007, based on 2006 annual fiscal year numbers) by the National Marrow Donor Program

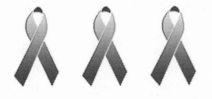

# Appendix F
# Conditions and Complications
# I Encountered

Leukemia
  AML
  Granulocytic sarcoma
Autonomic neuropathy
Cataracts in both eyes
Concussions (three)
Diabetes—steroid induced
GVHD (stomach, liver, eyes, and lungs)
Hearing loss
Heart-related
  Atrial fibrillation
  Cardiomyopathy
  Congestive heart failure
High/low blood pressure
Hydrocephalus
Hygromas
Lung-related
  Bronchiolitis obliterans

GVHD

Osteoporosis

   Broken hip

   Fractured tibia

Peripheral neuropathy

Pneumonia (several instances)

Pneumonitis

Septic shock

Testosterone deficiency

Tinnitus

Torn ligament in ankle

Typhlitis

Various infections/viruses (staph, fungal, cytomegalovirus, and *aspergillus*)

Vertebral fractures (eleven)

Vision loss

# CANCER GLOSSARY

During your journey through cancer, you will come across words and expressions that will not understand. What's more, you will find medical professionals using terms that are not common English. While not an exhaustive glossary, here are some words that you will likely come into contact with.

**ablate**. To remove by cutting.

**acute lymphocytic leukemia (ALL)**. Also known as **acute lymphoid leukemia** or **acute lymphoblastic leukemia**, a form of leukemia in which too many stem cells develop into a type of white blood cell called lymphocytes. The lymphocytes are not able to fight infection very well. Also, as the number of lymphocytes increases in the blood and bone marrow, there is less room for healthy white blood cells, red blood cells, and platelets. As a result, people with ALL develop red blood cell, platelet, and white cell deficiencies.

**acute myelogenous leukemia (AML)**. A form of leukemia that results from genetic damage to the DNA of cells. This cell damage results in: the uncontrolled growth of cells that are called "leukemic blasts." Leukemia cells are unable to do their usual work and can build up in the bone marrow and blood so there is less room for healthy white blood cells, red blood cells, and platelets. When this happens, infection, anemia, or easy bleeding may occur. The leukemia cells can spread outside the blood to other parts of the body, including the central nervous system (brain and spinal cord), skin, and gums. AML is not contagious nor is it inherited.

**adenocarcinoma.** Cancer that begins in cells that line certain internal organs and that have glandular (secretory) properties.

**adjuvant.** Serving to aid or contribute; involving the use of, or functioning as, a medical adjuvant (the action of a certain bacteria).

**adrenal gland.** The small gland found above each kidney, which secretes cortisone, adrenaline, aldosterone, and many other important hormones.

**ALL.** See **acute lymphocytic leukemia.**

**allogeneic bone marrow transplant.** A transplant in which marrow from a donor whose tissue type closely matches the patient's is used.

**alopecia.** Hair loss.

**AML.** See **acute myelogenous leukemia.**

**anesthesia.** Loss of feeling resulting from the administration of drugs or gases.

**angiogram.** An X-ray of blood vessels also called an arteriogram. For an angiogram, a dye is injected into an artery to outline the blood vessels on the X-ray picture.

**antibiotics.** Drugs used to treat infections.

**antibodies.** A large number of proteins that are produced normally after stimulation by an antigen and act specifically against the antigen in an immune response.

**anticoagulant**. A drug that reduces the blood's ability to clot.

**antigen**. A substance, foreign to the body that stimulates the production of antibodies by the immune system.

**aspiration**. Removal of fluid from a lump, often a cyst, with a needle.

**asymptomatic**. Not having any symptoms of a disease.

**autologous bone marrow transplant**. A transplant in which the marrow or cells from a patient is removed and then transfused back to the same person at a later date.

**atrial fibrillation**. A condition in which irregular, rapid beating of the atrial chambers of the heart conduct electricity in an abnormal manner so as to beat rapidly (possibly up to several hundred times per minute) and with an irregular rhythm.

**A-fib**. See **atrial fibrillation**.

**basal cell carcinoma**. The most common non-melanoma skin cancer. It begins in the lowest layer of the epidermis, called the basal cell layer. It usually develops on sun-exposed areas, especially the head and neck. Basal cell cancer is slow-growing and is not likely to spread to distant parts of the body.

**benign**. Not cancerous. Benign tumors do not spread to tissues around them or to other parts of the body.

**billiard**. Having to do with the liver, bile ducts, and/or gallbladder.

**biological therapy**. Treatment to stimulate or restore the ability of the immune system to fight infection and disease also called **immunotherapy**.

**biopsy**. The removal of cells or tissues for examination by a pathologist.

**blood count**. The amount of white cells, red cells, and platelets in a sample of blood drawn from a patient's body.

**bone marrow transplantation**. A procedure in which doctors replace marrow destroyed by treatment with high doses of anti-cancer drugs or radiation. The replacement marrow may be taken from the patient before treatment or may be donated by another person.

**bone marrow**. The soft inner part of large bones that produces blood cells.

**bone scan**. A test to determine if there is any sign of cancer in the bones.

**brachytherapy**. A form of internal radiation treatment given by placing radioactive material directly into the tumor or close to it.

**brain scan**. An imaging method used to find anything abnormal in the brain, including brain cancer and cancer that has spread to the brain from other places in the body.

**breast cancer**. Cancer that starts in the breast.

**bronchiolitis obliterans**. A disease of the lungs in which the bronchioles are plugged.

**bronchoscopy**. Examination of the bronchi using a flexible, lighted tube called a bronchoscope

**calcifications**. Tiny calcium deposits within the breast, singly or in clusters, often found by mammography.

**cancer**. A term for diseases in which abnormal cells divide without control.

**carcinogen**. A substance or agent that is known to cause cancer.

**carcinogenesis**. The process by which normal cells are transformed into cancer cells.

**carcinoma**. Cancer that begins in the skin or in tissues that line or cover internal organs.

**carcinoma in situ**. Cancer that involves only the tissue in which it began; it has not spread to other tissues.

**catheter**. A thin plastic tube that is placed in a vein and provides a pathway for drugs, nutrients, or blood products. Blood samples also can be removed through the catheter.

**cell**. The smallest living unit. All living tissue is composed of cells.

**central line**. A type of catheter used to remove fluids from or provide fluids to the body.

**chemotherapy**. The use of chemical agents or anticancer drugs in the treatment or control of disease.

**chromosome**. A macromolecule of DNA that carries the genes, which are the basic units of heredity. Humans have twenty-three pairs of chromosomes, one member of each pair from the mother, the other from the father. Each chromosome can contain hundreds or thousands of individual genes.

**chronic lymphocytic leukemia (CLL)**. A type of leukemia that results from an acquired injury to the DNA of a single cell in the bone marrow that is not present at birth. The change in the cell's DNA results in the uncontrolled growth of CLL cells in the marrow, leading to an increased concentration in the blood. The lymphocytes in CLL, B lymphocytes, T lymphocytes, and natural killer cells are not able to fight infection very well. Also, as the amount of lymphocytes increases in the blood and bone marrow, there is less room for healthy white blood cells, red blood cells, and platelets. This may result in infection, anemia, and easy bleeding.

**chronic myelogenous leukemia (CML)**. A form of leukemia that results from an acquired injury to the DNA of a stem cell in the marrow and is not present at birth. As a result of this DNA change, the individual experiences an uncontrolled growth of white blood cells. Unlike AML, chronic myelogenous leukemia permits the development of normally-functioning white blood cells. This important distinction from acute leukemia accounts for the less severe early course of the disease.

**clinical trial**. A research study that involves human volunteers with specific health conditions. A trial allows the examination of a proposed drug or therapy in a controlled environment to determine its safety and effectiveness in treating patients with certain conditions.

**CLL**. See **chronic lymphocytic leukemia**.

**CML**. See **chronic myelogenous leukemia**.

**colectomy**. An operation to remove all or part of the colon.

**colon**. The long, coiled, tube-like organ that removes water from digested food.

**colonoscope**. A flexible, lighted instrument used to view the inside of the colon

**colonoscopy**. An examination in which the doctor looks at the colon through a colonoscope.

**colony-stimulating factors**. Substances that stimulate the production of blood cells.

**colostomy**. An opening created by a surgeon into the colon from the outside of the body. A colostomy provides a new path for waste material to leave the body after part of the colon has been removed.

**Comprehensive Cancer Center**. A designation by the National Cancer Institute (NCI) indicating that a facility has fulfilled of criteria related to research and public information, education, and outreach activities.

**congestive heart failure (CHF)**. A condition in which the heart muscle is not able to pump enough blood to satisfy the metabolic needs of the tissues. Heart failure may be due to a primary disease of the heart muscle, which is called cardiomyopathy, or it may be secondary to diseases that affect the heart muscle such as hypertension, coronary heart disease, or various diseases of the heart valves.

**consolidation**. A term that refers to the period of chemotherapy after normal induction chemotherapy when a more intensive round of chemotherapy is given in order to achieve a remission.

**continence**. The ability to retain a bodily discharge (urine or fecal) voluntarily.

**core biopsy**. The removal of a tissue sample with a needle for examination under a microscope.

**CT or CAT scan**. Detailed pictures of areas of the body created by a computer linked to an X-ray machine. CT is an acronym for **computed tomography**, and CAT is an acronym for **computed axial tomography**.

**cyst**. A closed sac or capsule usually filled with fluid or semisolid material.

**cystectomy**. Surgery to remove all or part of the bladder.

**cystoscope**. An instrument that allows the doctor to see inside the bladder and remove tissue samples or small tumors.

**cystoscopy**. Examination of the bladder with an instrument called a cystoscope.

**cytology**. The branch of science that deals with the structure and function of cells. Cytology also refers to tests to diagnose cancer and other diseases by examination of cells under the microscope.

**cytotoxic**. Chemicals that are directly toxic to cells, preventing their reproduction or growth. Cytotoxic agents can, as a side effect, damage healthy, noncancerous tissues, or organs that have a high proportion of actively dividing cells—for example, bone marrow, or hair follicles. These side effects limit the amount and frequency of drug administration.

**diabetes**. A disease that results from the body's inability to regulate glucose (sugar) levels.

**digital rectal exam**. An exam to detect rectal cancer.

**DNA (deoxyribonucleic acid)**. A substance containing genetic information that is found inside the center (nucleus) of cells. DNA determines what features a person inherits from his or her parents, such as blood type, hair color, eye color, and other characteristics.

**duct**. A tube in the breast through which body fluids pass. Cancer that begins in a duct is called ductal carcinoma.

**dysplasia**. Abnormal cells that are not cancerous.

**edema**. Swelling caused by a collection of fluid in the soft tissues.

**ejection fraction**. The fraction of blood pumped out of a ventricle with each heart beat.

**endoscopy**. A procedure in which the doctor looks inside the body through a lighted tube called an endoscope.

**epidemiology**. The study of diseases in populations by collecting and analyzing statistical data.

**estrogen**. A female sex hormone produced primarily by the ovaries and in smaller amounts by the adrenal cortex.

**etiology**. The cause or origin of disease.

**Ewing's sarcoma**. A bone cancer that forms in the middle of large bones. Ewing's sarcoma most often affects the hip bones and the bones of the upper arm and thigh.

**excision biopsy**. A surgical procedure in which an entire lump or suspicious area is removed for diagnosis. The tissue is then examined under a microscope.

**fine-needle aspiration**. The removal of tissue or fluid with a needle for examination under a microscope also called **needle biopsy**.

**gamma rays**. Forms of electromagnetic radiation that are similar to X-rays but that come from a different radioactive source.

**gastroenterologist**. A doctor who specializes in diseases of the digestive (gastrointestinal) tract.

**gastrointestinal**. Pertaining to the stomach and intestines. The major sub sites of GI cancer are stomach/esophagus, colorectal, and hepatobiliary.

**gene therapy**. Treatment that alters a gene. In studies of gene therapy for cancer, researchers are trying to improve the body's natural ability to fight the disease or to make the cancer cells more sensitive to other kinds of therapy.

**gene**. A segment of DNA that contains information on hereditary characteristics such as hair color, eye color, and height, as well as susceptibility to certain diseases.

**genetics**. A branch of biology that deals with the hereditary and variation of organisms. Anything that is genetic is inherited and having to do with information that is passed from parents to offspring through genes in sperm and egg cells.

**genitourinary**. The parts of the body that play a role in the reproduction and the urinary systems.

**genitourinary tract**. The system of organs concerned with the production and excretion of urine.

**graft-versus-host disease (GVH) or (GVHD)**. A disorder that can occur following an allogeneic transplant. With GVHD, the newly transplanted cells fight against cells and organs from the host cells and result in symptoms generally related to the skin, eyes, intestines, liver, and lungs. It can be a serious problem and be either an acute or chronic condition for the patient.

**GVH**. See **graft-versus-host disease**.

**GVHD**. See **graft-versus-host disease**

**gynecologic**. Having to do with the female reproductive tract (including the cervix, endometrial, fallopian tubes, ovaries, uterus, and vagina). Gynecologic oncology concerns endometrial, ovarian, uterine, and cervical cancer.

**hematocrit**. The percentage of red blood cells.

**hematologist**. A doctor who specializes in diseases of the blood and blood-forming tissues.

**hematology**. Medical specialty in treating blood disorders.

**hematoma**. A collection of blood outside a blood vessel caused by a leak or an injury.

**hemoglobin**. The <u>iron</u>-containing <u>oxygen</u> protein in the <u>red blood cells</u>.

**hemorrhage**. To lose of blood through heavy, uncontrolled bleeding.

**heparin**. A drug that decreases the clotting tendency of blood.

**hepatic** vein. Any of the veins that carry the blood received from the hepatic artery and from the hepatic portal vein away from the liver.

**hepatobiliary**. Pertaining to the liver and the bile or the billiard ducts.

**hepatocellular** carcinoma. A type of adenocarcinoma, the most common type of liver tumor.

**hickman**. A type of catheter used to remove fluids from or provide fluids to the body.

**Hodgkin's disease**. A type of cancer that affects the lymphatic system.

**hormonal therapies**. Therapeutic use of hormones for the treatment of cancer in which the growth of certain cancers (such as prostate and breast cancer) is slowed or stopped by the administering of synthetic hormones or other drugs to block the body's natural hormones.

**hormone**. A chemical substance produced by glands in the body that enters the bloodstream and causes effects in other tissues.

**human leukocyte antigen (HLA) system**. The name of the human major histocompatibility complex that encodes cell-surface antigen-presenting proteins. The chance of two individuals having identical HLA molecules is very low, except for among siblings, who have a 25 percent chance of being HLA-identical. HLA matching is important in bone marrow transplanting.

**hysterectomy**. Surgery to remove the uterus and, sometimes, the cervix. When the uterus and part or the entire cervix is removed, it is called a total hysterectomy. When only the uterus is removed, it is called a partial hysterectomy.

**immune system**. A complex system by which the body is able to protect itself from foreign invaders.

**immunology**. The study of how the body resists infection and certain other diseases.

**immunosuppression**. A state in which the ability of the body's immune system to respond is decreased.

**immunotherapy**. Treatment to stimulate or restore the ability of the immune system to fight infections and other diseases, which is also used to lessen certain side effects that may be caused by cancer treatment.

**impotence**. An abnormal physical or psychological state of a male characterized by the inability to copulate because of failure to have or maintain an erection.

**incision biopsy**. A surgical procedure in which a portion of a lump or suspicious area is removed for diagnosis. The tissue is then examined under a microscope.

**induction**. The initial phases of chemotherapy.

**in situ**. A term that refers to tumors that haven't grown beyond their site of origin.

**intraoperative**. Occurring, carried out, or encountered in the course of surgery.

**intrathecal chemotherapy**. Injection of anticancer drugs into the cerebrospinal fluid.

**intravenous (IV)**. Administration of a drug directly into a vein.

**invasive ductal carcinoma**. A cancer that starts in the milk passages (ducts) of the breast and then breaks through the duct wall, where it invades the fatty tissue of the breast.

**invasive lobular carcinoma**. A cancer that starts in the milk-producing glands (lobules) of the breast and then breaks through the lobule walls to invade the nearby fatty tissue.

**Kaposi's sarcoma**. A type of cancer characterized by the abnormal growth of blood vessels that develop into skin lesions or occur internally.

**laryngectomy**. Surgery to remove the voice box (larynx), usually because of cancer.

**lesion**. (1) A change in body tissue (2) a term that is sometimes used as another word for tumor.

**leukemia**. Cancer that starts in blood-forming tissue such as the bone marrow and causes large numbers of abnormal blood cells to be produced and enter the bloodstream.

**leukocytosis**. Having more than the usual number of white blood cells.

**leukopenia**. Decrease in the white blood cell count, often a side effect of chemotherapy.

**linear accelerator**. A machine used in radiation therapy to treat cancer.

**lobectomy**. Surgery to remove a lobe of an organ, usually the lung.

**low microbial diet**. A special diet provided to patients whose immune systems are compromised and need a special diet. See Appendix D for details.

**lumpectomy**. Surgery to remove a lump and a small margin of normal tissue surrounding it.

**lymph**. The almost colorless fluid that bathes body cells and contains cells that help fight infection.

**lymph nodes**. Any of the rounded masses of lymphoid tissue surrounded by a capsule of connective tissue that occur in association with the lymphatic vessels.

**lymphatic system**. The lymph nodes, spleen, and thymus—which produce and store infection-fighting cells—and the network of channels that carry lymph fluid.

**lymphedema.** A complication that sometimes happens after breast cancer treatments. Swelling in the arm is caused by excess lymph fluid that collects after lymph nodes and vessels are removed by surgery or treated by radiation.

**lymphocytes.** White blood cells critical to the immune system's defense against disease organisms in the body, including cancer cells.

**lymphoma.** A cancer that originates in the body's lymphatic tissues, primarily the lymph nodes, or the lymph tissue of such organs as the stomach, small intestine, or bone.

**magnetic resonance imaging (MRI).** A method of taking pictures of the inside of the body. Instead of using X-rays, MRI uses a powerful magnet and transmits radio waves through the body.

**malignancy.** The quality or state of being cancerous.

**mammogram.** An X-ray of the breast.

**mastectomy.** Surgery to remove the breast (or as much of the breast tissue as possible).

**matched unrelated donor (MUD).** A person whose HLA system sufficiently matches that of a patient in need of an allogeneic transplant who is not related to the patient.

**melanoma.** A form of skin cancer that produce pigment. Melanoma usually begins in a mole.

**mesothelioma.** A benign (noncancerous) or malignant (cancerous) tumor affecting the lining of the chest or abdomen. Exposure to asbestos particles in the air increases the risk of developing malignant mesothelioma.

**metastasis.** Spread of cancer to another organ, usually through the bloodstream.

**modality.** A method of treatment. For example, surgery and chemotherapy are treatment modalities.

**molecular biology.** A branch of biology dealing with the physicochemical organization of living matter.

**monoclonal antibodies.** Substances that can locate and bind to cancer cells wherever they are in the body. Monoclonal antibodies can be used alone or used to deliver drugs, toxins, or radioactive material directly to the tumor cells.

**morbidity.** A measure of the new cases of a disease in a population; the number of people who have a disease.

**mortality.** A measure of the rate of death from a disease within a given population.

**mucinous carcinoma.** A type of carcinoma that is formed by mucus-producing cancer cells.

**mucositis.** Inflammation of a mucous membrane such as the lining of the mouth.

**multiple gated acquisition (MUGA) scan.** A scan in which the function of the heart is assessed. It produces a moving image of the beating heart, and from this image several important features can be determined about the health of the cardiac ventricles (the heart's major pumping chambers).

**multiple myeloma.** Cancer that begins in the cells of the immune system.

**nadir.** Period of time following chemotherapy treatment when blood counts generally are at their lowest levels and patients are at greatest risk of developing infection and other blood-related side effects.

**National Cancer Institute (NCI).** A component of the National Institutes of Health (NIH). The NCI coordinates the National

Cancer Program, which conducts and supports research, training, health information dissemination, and other programs with respect to the causes, diagnoses, prevention, and treatment of cancer; the rehabilitation from cancer; and the continuing care of cancer patients and the families of cancer patients.

**necrosis.** Dead tissue.

**needle biopsy.** The removal of tissue or fluid with a needle for examination under a microscope. See also fine-needle aspiration.

**neoplasm.** An abnormal growth (tumor) that starts from a single altered cell; a neoplasm may be benign or malignant. Cancer is a malignant neoplasm.

**nephrectomy.** Surgery to remove a kidney or part of a kidney.

**neurooncology.** Specialty concerning the diagnosis and treatment of brain tumors and other tumors of the nervous system.

**neutropenia.** A condition in which the patient has less than the normal number of neutrophils, a type of white blood cell that helps to defend against bacterial infections.

**neutrophils.** White blood cells that fight bacterial infection.

**nodule.** A small, solid lump that can be located by touch. Nodule is sometimes used to refer to a small tumor seen on X-ray.

**non-Hodgkin's lymphoma.** A cancer of the lymphatic system.

**oncogenes.** Genes that promote cell growth and multiplication. These genes are normally present in all cells, but oncogenes may undergo changes that activate them, causing cells to grow too quickly and form tumors.

**oncologist.** A doctor who specializes in treating cancer. Some oncologists specialize in a particular type of cancer treatment. For example, a radiation oncologist specializes in treating cancer with radiation.

**oncology**. The branch of medicine that studies cancer or malignant diseases.

**oophorectomy**. Surgery to remove the ovaries.

**orchiectomy**. Surgery to remove the testicles.

**osteoporosis**. A disease that weakens bones, increasing the risk of sudden and unexpected fractures. Literally meaning "porous bone," osteoporosis results in an increased loss of bone mass and strength. The disease often progresses without any symptoms or pain.

**ostomy**. A general term meaning an opening, especially one made by surgery.

**palliative therapy**. A treatment that may relieve symptoms without curing the disease.

**pancreatectomy**. Surgery to remove the pancreas.

**papillary**. Having cancer cells arranged in tiny, finger-like projections.

**pathologist**. a physician who interprets and analyzes the changes caused by disease in tissues and body fluids.

**peripheral blood stem cell transplant (PBSCT)**. A method for replacing bone marrow destroyed by cancer treatment.

**petechiae**. Small hemorrhages of the tiny blood vessels found just below the skin surface. Petechiae often result from a low platelet count and always disappear when the platelet count rises again.

**pharmacotherapy**. The treatment of a disease with drugs.

**PICC Line**. A type of catheter used to remove fluids from or provide fluids to the body. Short for Peripherally inserted central catheter.

**platelets**. Blood cells that seal off injuries and prevent excessive bleeding without clotting.

**polyp**. A mass of tissue that develops on the inside wall of a hollow organ such as the colon.

**positron emission tomography (PET) scan**. A scan in which an image of the body is created, with the injection of a very low dose of a radioactive form of a substance such as glucose, in order to find the presence of cancer.

**posterior**. Laterally situated at or toward the hinder end of the body; lying at or extending toward the right or left side of the body.

**primary site**. The place where cancer begins. Primary cancer is usually named after the organ in which it starts. For example, cancer that starts in the breast is always breast cancer even if it spreads (metastasizes) to other organs such as bones or lungs.

**prognosis**. Expected or probable outcome.

**prostate gland**. A gland in the male reproductive system just below the bladder. The prostrate gland surrounds part of the urethra, the canal that empties the bladder.

**prostate specific antigen (PSA)**. A PSA test is used to help find prostate cancer as well as to monitor the results of treatment.

**prostatectomy**. An operation to remove part or the entire prostate. Radical (or total) prostatectomy is the removal of the entire prostate and some of the tissue around it.

**protocol**. A formal outline or plan, such as a description of what treatments a patient will receive and exactly when each should be given.

**radiation oncologist**. A specialist in utilizing radiation as a means of cancer treatment.

**radiation therapy**. Treatment with high-energy rays (such as X-rays) to kill or shrink cancer cells. The radiation may come from outside of the body (external radiation) or from radioactive materials placed directly in the tumor (internal or implant radiation). Radiation therapy may be used to reduce the size of a cancer before surgery, to destroy any remaining cancer cells after surgery, or, in some cases, as the main treatment.

**radical cystectomy**. Surgery to remove the bladder as well as nearby tissues and organs.

**radical hysterectomy**. Surgery to remove the uterus, cervix, and part of the vagina. The ovaries, fallopian tubes, and nearby lymph nodes may also be removed.

**radical lymph node dissection**. A surgical procedure to remove most or all of the lymph nodes that drain lymph from the area around a tumor. The lymph nodes are then examined under a microscope to see if cancer cells have spread to them.

**radical mastectomy**. Surgery for breast cancer in which the breast, chest muscles, and all of the lymph nodes under the arm are removed.

**radioactive implant**. A source of high-dose radiation that is placed directly into or around a tumor to kill the cancer cells.

**radio-isotope bone scan**. A diagnostic procedure in which a harmless amount of radioactive chemical is injected into the bloodstream and concentrates in cancer cells.

**radiologist**. A physician with special training in reading diagnostic X-rays and performing specialized X-ray procedures.

**radiotherapy**. The treatment of disease by radiation.

**rectum**. The last five to six inches of the colon leading to the outside of the body.

**recurrence.** Return of cancer after its apparent complete disappearance.

**red cells.** Cells produced by bone marrow that circulate in the blood and carry oxygen to all parts of the body.

**relapse.** Reappearance of cancer after a disease-free period.

**remission.** Disappearance of detectable disease. Remission is not a cure.

**renal cell carcinoma.** A malignant tumor relating to the kidneys.

**sarcoma.** Cancer that begins in bone, cartilage, fat, muscle, blood vessels, or other connective or supportive tissue.

**secondary tumor.** A tumor that forms as a result of spread (metastasis) of cancer from the place where it started.

**sigmoidoscope.** A lighted instrument used to view the inside of the lower colon.

**sigmoidoscopy.** An examination of the rectum and lower colon using a sigmoidoscope.

**spinal tap.** A procedure in which a thin needle is placed in the spinal canal to withdraw a small amount of spinal fluid or to get medicine into the central nervous system through the spinal fluid.

**squamous cell carcinoma.** Cancer that begins in the non-glandular cells, for example, the skin.

**staging.** The process of learning whether cancer has spread from its original site to another part of the body.

**steroids.** Drugs used to relieve swelling and inflammation

**stoma.** (1) Any of various small simple openings. (2) An artificial permanent opening in the abdominal wall made in surgical procedures (a colostomy).

**syngeneic transplant**. A transplant received from an identical twin.

**systemic disease**. In cancer, a term that means that the tumor that originated in one place has spread to distant organs or structures.

**thrombocytopenia**. A decrease in the number of platelets in the blood, which can be a side effect of chemotherapy.

**T lymphocytes or T cells**. White blood cells made in the thymus gland. T cells produce lymphokines and play a large role in the immune response against viruses, transplanted organs and tissues, and cancer cells.

**total body irradiation** (TBI). Radiation treatment that is given to a patient's entire body.

**translational research**. The clinical application of scientific medical research, from the lab to the bedside.

**tumor**. An abnormal mass of tissue that is not inflammatory, arises from cells of preexistent tissue, and serves no useful purpose. A tumor results when cells divide more than they should or do not die when they should.

**typhlitis**. An inflammation of the abdomen, which can quickly spread to other areas. Tyhplitis often results in perforation of the abdomen and can have a high mortality rate.

**ultrasound**. A diagnostic procedure that bounces high-frequency sound waves off tissues and changes the echoes into pictures.

**urologic oncology**. The study of tumors of or relating to the urinary tract.

**vein**. A blood vessel that carries blood from the tissues toward the heart and lungs.

**viruses.** Tiny parasites that cause infectious disease. Viruses can only divide and multiply in living cells.

**Whipple procedure.** Surgery used to treat pancreatic cancer.

**white blood cells.** Cells produced by the bone marrow and lymph nodes that help the body fight infection.

**X-ray.** High-energy radiation used in low doses to diagnose diseases and in high doses to treat cancers.

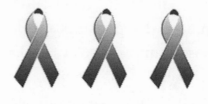

# About the Author

Rusty Hammer was diagnosed with a rare form of an aggressive leukemia in 2003. Having survived, he battles significant side and after effects—seeking a cure that has been worse than the disease. His life story and his battle against cancer will amaze and engage you.

Rusty grew up in Campbell, California. He became involved in politics at a very young age; at age eighteen, he became the youngest elected official then in U.S. history and, at twenty-one, he was the youngest mayor in U.S. history at the time. Following his political career, Rusty had a successful business career that culminated in his service as a corporate CEO of a thousand-employee energy and environmental company.

After leaving the private sector, he took a position as president and chief executive officer of the Sacramento Metropolitan Chamber of Commerce. After completing a turnaround of that organization, he was recruited to the same position at the Los Angeles Area Chamber of Commerce where, as the leading spokesperson and representative for the business community in the nation's second largest business region, he turned the chamber into a dynamic and aggressive organization at the forefront of public policy initiatives in California.

It was while in Los Angeles that Rusty was diagnosed with a rare form of leukemia and, as a result, was forced to retire from his duties due to the disabling nature of his illness, although he continues to work with the chamber in a limited capacity.

He currently serves as a member of the Board of Directors of the National Marrow Donor Program and its strategic planning committee.

He and his wife, Pamela, live in San Jose, California, and their children, Gerald and Jennifer (twenty-six-year-old twins) live in Southern California.

978-0-595-44735-0
0-595-44735-X

Made in the USA